Great Diabetic Desserts & Sweets

Karin Cadwell, Ph.D., R.N.
& Edith White, M.Ed.

Foreword by John F. Coughlin, M.D., Ph.D.
Medical Director, Joslin Diabetes Center / Falmouth

Sterling Publishing Co., Inc.   New York

We want to thank Anna Cadwell, Ruth Maas McIlhenny, Kirstin Cadwell, Joanne McIlhenny, and Annette Carpenter, who contributed their time and talent to the production of this book. Without their efforts, this project could not have been completed.

We also want to thank our friends and family, diabetic and not, for all their help and encouragement.

Because our idea was to produce a cookbook of diabetic desserts that diabetics and non-diabetics would both love, virtually everyone we knew became a taste tester. We brought food to all kinds of occasions, from square dances to church socials to birthday parties. Family members and friends became accustomed to several desserts at lunch and dinner. We think we have accomplished our goal and that your friends and family members, diabetic and not, will love these desserts.

Library of Congress Cataloging-in-Publication Data

Cadwell, Karin.
    Great diabetic desserts & sweets / by Karin Cadwell & Edith White ;
foreword by John F. Coughlin.
        p. cm.
    Includes index.
    ISBN 0-8069-3845-5
    1. Diabetes—Diet therapy—Recipes. 2. Desserts. I. White, Edith.
RC662.C316   1995
641.5'6314—dc20   95-20036
                                                                         CIP

10 9 8 7 6 5 4 3 2 1
Published by Sterling Publishing Company, Inc.
387 Park Avenue South, New York, N.Y. 10016
© 1995 by Karin Cadwell and Edith White
Distributed in Canada by Sterling Publishing
C/o Canadian Manda Group, One Atlantic Avenue, Suite 105
Toronto, Ontario, Canada M6K 3E7
Distributed in Great Britain and Europe by Cassell PLC
Wellington House, 125 Strand, London WC2R 0BB, England
Distributed in Australia by Capricorn Link (Australia) Pty Ltd.
P.O. Box 6651, Baulkham Hills, Business Centre, NSW 2153, Australia
Manufactured in the United States of America
All rights reserved

Sterling ISBN 0-8069-3845-5

Contents

Foreword

Many patients who are diabetic or who for other reasons have problems controlling their blood pressure, blood sugar levels, cholesterol, or weight have come to my office looking for solutions to their health problems. Most of them have already tried a variety of "quick fix" schemes and have either given up all hope of living a so-called "normal" life or are still searching for a magic panacea. They fear being put on the dreaded "diet," considering it to be more of a punishment than a cure. They couldn't be more wrong.

Unlike short-term crash diets, which have proven to be ineffective in the long run, changes in eating habits are a positive step towards a healthier, happier lifestyle. They make you look and feel better and significantly reduce the risk of a variety of illnesses. Far from being a punishment, they reap innumerable rewards. For example, a recent large nationwide study indicated that when blood sugars were lowered, people with type I diabetes reduced diabetic eye complications by 54 to 76 percent, kidney complications by 39 to 54 percent, and nerve problems by 60 percent.

Let's not forget that a diet that's good for someone with diabetes is good for someone with a heart condition, a cholesterol problem, or a weight problem. In fact, it's just plain good for anyone!

As Karin Cadwell and Edith White prove in this remarkable cookbook, choosing a healthier eating plan does not mean you have to sacrifice taste, satisfaction, or fun. Packed with mouth-watering desserts, this volume is a powerful tool to help anyone, diabetic or not, in developing a healthier way of living. The recipes are easy to follow, and yield delicious, wholesome results that the whole family will love.

Enjoy!

John F. Coughlin, M.D., Ph.D.
Medical Director
Joslin Diabetes Center/Falmouth

CHAPTER ONE

Our Desserts Are Good Enough for Everyone!

We offer this cookbook as a help to people with diabetes, people who want to enjoy delicious desserts while keeping their blood sugar under control. Like many others, we were impressed by the results of the 1993 Diabetes Control & Complication Trial: People who kept their blood sugar as close to normal as possible reduced the risk of diabetic eye disease by 76%, kidney disease by 35–56%, and nerve damage by 60%.

If you are diabetic, your physician probably reminds you of the importance of controlling your blood sugar. What we offer is just a cookbook, not a book on diabetes. Individual advice from your physician on managing your diabetes must come before anything we say. Individualized diet advice from your dietitian or diabetic educator also comes before anything we say.

Neither of us is diabetic, although we have friends and family members with diabetes, people for whom we cook. Karin remembers growing up and hearing how her grandmother's cooking kept her diabetic husband in good health. She was a cordon bleu chef who improvised all kinds of recipes for her husband. We are fortunate enough to share her legacy of recipes. In the last few years, almost all of Edith's cooking has been for a dear friend who happens to be diabetic.

Our philosophy is that recipes should be so delicious that everyone in the family is served the same dessert. The idea of serving the same dish to everyone began years ago with cooking classes and a book we did for people who needed to restrict their sodium or salt. We noticed that in some families everyone was served "regular" (high-sodium) tasty foods, everyone except the person on the special diet, who was served rather unpalatable "low sodium" foods. In other families where everyone was served the same low-sodium foods, an effort was made to see that the food was truly delicious. Our experience has been overwhelmingly the same: People make more of an effort to see that foods are delicious when everyone eats the same thing.

We believe that it is quite feasible to serve desserts that are good for diabetics and acceptable to other people too. We offer here a collection of recipes with little or no sugar or other concentrated sweets, and with as little fat as possible. We have been troubled by real-life scenes in which everyone is served some tempting dessert—everyone, that is, except the diabetic. "We're having chocolate cake and ice cream tonight...except for Tom. (He's diabetic.) Here's your apple, Tom."

What's wrong with this scene? First of all, it's not very considerate of Tom's feelings. Who among us wants to hear the people closest to us remind us that we are different? Second, we have seen chocolate cakes and such lead diabetic friends off their diets. We can add a third reason for serving the same dessert to everyone: Those of us who are fortunate enough not to have diabetes still have coronary arteries. We do not need the saturated fat, cholesterol, and calories associated with classic dessert ingredients (heavy cream, chocolate, cream cheese, egg yolks).

In our recipes we make much use of cocoa, nonfat cream cheese, skim milk, nonfat ricotta cheese, nonfat cottage cheese, and egg whites or egg substitutes. If any non-diabetic cooks reading this introduction need one more reason to serve everyone the same dessert, here it is: People who are related to a diabetic are at a higher genetic risk for developing diabetes themselves as they get older. People with a genetic predisposition to diabetes are unwise to let themselves become overweight. Although we non-diabetics may be able to better tolerate concentrated sweets, we don't need them. Getting into the habit of stocking our kitchens with low-calorie, low-fat, low-sugar ingredients can make it easier to keep the extra pounds off.

What About Fats?

On the issue of which fats to buy, there may not be a simple answer. Butter or margarine? Both have problems. The problems with butter have been well publicized: Butter has saturated fat and cholesterol. But recently margarine has come under increasing attack. British medical experts in November 1994 issued a warning against margarine's trans fatty acids and against hydrogenated polyunsaturated fats. Some researchers have linked vegetable oils with an increased risk of cardiovascular heart disease.

Is Margarine Healthier Than Butter?

Some medical and nutritional experts would say that it is, while others disagree. Your information may vary, depending on what country you live in. Some people use neither butter nor margarine. They use olive oil in cooking. They may also use a non-stick cooking spray. We have a friend who keeps a little sign to himself on his toaster: "Use jelly, stupid." In our recipes we say "margarine or butter." You decide after talking to your physician, dietitian, or diabetic educator. We call for as little fat as possible. But for cookies or flour-based pie crust, either use a little fat or just don't make the recipe. We suggest saving richer confections that require more than one fat exchange for special occasions, for everyone.

Honest Reading of Dietary Information

In our recipes we tell you, among other things, how many calories and grams of fat a recipe has, and what the diabetic exchanges are per serving. Please be aware, however, that stated portions in all recipes today, ours included, are for very small portions. Portion sizes have been standardized;

these standard portions are smaller than what many people eat in real life. A serving of cake is listed as one-twelfth or even one-twentieth of the cake. "Nice" portions are likely to be twice that size. If you eat a generous portion, you need to double (or sometimes triple) the nutritional values and diabetic exchanges.

Some Recipes Are Healthier Than Others

In this cookbook, we give you a range of recipes. Fresh fruit is a classic healthy dessert. Many people with diabetes make it a habit to save one fruit exchange to have as their dessert. Many of our fruit-based recipes cost few calories and one fruit exchange. We also offer recipes for richer desserts that cost more calories and exchanges, in which case you may need to plan your eating to save enough fat and starch exchanges for dessert.

Desserts Are Expected to Taste Sweet

Human beings like the natural sweet taste of sugar (sucrose), honey, maple syrup, molasses, corn syrup, etc. These are all caloric sweeteners. We'll discuss non-caloric sweeteners a little later. Sugar is not the only caloric sweetener that can raise your blood sugar. Labels on food products often brag that they contain no sugar. But they may contain other ingredients that raise your blood sugar. Some "no sugar" cookbooks make great use of sweet fruit juice concentrates. Frozen grape juice concentrate adds a nice, sweet taste to foods, but many diabetics who check their blood sugar find it acts just like sugar. That's why it gives such a nice, sweet taste. Apple juice concentrate also adds sweetness.

You will need to test your own blood sugar to see how your body reacts.

Fructose is a fruit sugar; it can be found in the "diet" section of most large food stores. Some diabetics whose blood sugar is under good control find that fructose causes less of a blood sugar rise than sucrose. Also, since it is sweeter, you can use less in cooking. But we know diabetics in good control who find that fructose plays havoc with their blood sugar. When you test your blood sugar, you will learn how fructose or fruit juice concentrates affect you as an individual.

Diabetics were traditionally told to avoid sugar completely. But more recently researchers have found that diabetics can tolerate small amounts of sugar when they take it in at the same time as other foods.

Some recipes call for a very small amount of sugar. In cake recipes, for example, sugar does more than just add sweetness. Its bulk is necessary for the cake to rise up and be light and tender and, well, cakelike. A cake made with no sugar or with a relative like fructose will not have the tenderness, color, or texture of cake. One-twelfth of a cake made with a very small amount of sugar contains very little sugar indeed.

9

Sorbitol and its relative mannitol are caloric sweeteners that are used in manufacturing commercial products. Sorbitol is found in some "diabetic" products such as candy bars. Sorbitol has distinct drawbacks: First, it gives many people diarrhea. Secondly, it has calories. Third, its presence in a confection often makes it necessary to add fat for creaminess. So a product with sorbitol is not necessarily good for a person with diabetes.

You can now buy many jelly substitutes or fruit spreads made without sugar. Some are made with saccharin. With others, the first ingredient listed may be a sweet juice concentrate, which can raise your blood sugar. Read carefully all labels that brag about having no sugar added. Ask your dietitian or diabetic educator about any products that confuse you. And, of course, test your blood sugar to know how different products affect you.

Alcohol is another ingredient where professional advice is needed. Although people with diabetes traditionally have been advised not to drink at all, newer research says that some can drink limited amounts of non-sweet drinks at the same time that other foods are eaten. In a few recipes we have used very small amounts of liqueurs to add flavor to cooked dishes. The longer the cooking, the more alcohol cooks out, leaving just a nice flavor.

Non-Caloric Sweeteners

As they say on TV, can we talk? Can we admit that sugar substitutes can taste awful? Many people find the taste of saccharin bitter. We didn't find anyone, diabetic or not, who liked the taste of saccharin brown sugar substitute. It's simple enough for a recipe to call for brown sugar substitute but that doesn't mean the finished dish will taste the same as it would with brown sugar.

The three major sugar substitutes available in the United States are saccharin (Sweet'n Low®, Sugar Twin®, Sprinkle Sweet®), aspartame (Equal®, Equal Measure®, NutraSweet® or NutraSweet Spoonful®), and acesulfame-K (Sweet One®). The subject of sugar substitutes is quite confusing because of all the brand names and different formulations. We offer two charts. The first will help you know which ingredient our recipes call for without using brand names. It will also help you in shopping. The second chart will help you adapt your old recipes to the use of artificial sweeteners.

In our recipes we call for specific non-caloric sweeteners. We have found that in many cases a particular one works better than the others for specific recipes. Note carefully whether a recipe (ours or anyone else's) calls for a product that is substituted cup for cup with sugar. We use the phrase "measures-like-sugar saccharin" to refer to products such as Sugar Twin® that are substituted, cup for cup with sugar. We use the phrase "measures-like-sugar aspartame" to refer to products such as NutraSweet Spoonful®. Most artificial sweetener products, however, are formulated to require much smaller amounts. We use the words "saccharin," "aspartame," or "acesulfame-K" for these concentrated products.

Amount of Artificial Sweeteners to Substitute for Sugar

Sugar	Acesulfame-K	Aspartame	Saccharin
2 t	1 pkt	1 pkt or ¼ t	1 pkt or ⅕ t
1 T	1¼ pkt	1½ pkt or ½ t	1⅓ pkt or ⅓ t
¼ cup	3 pkt	6 pkt or 1¾ t	3 pkt or 1⅙ t
⅓ cup	4 pkt	8 pkt or 2½ t	4 pkt or 1¼ t
½ cup	6 pkt	12 pkt or 3½ t	6 pkt or 2 t
⅔ cup	8 pkt	16 pkt or 5 t	8 pkt or 2½ t
¾ cup	9 pkt	18 pkt or 5¼ t	9 pkt or 3½ t
1 cup	12 pkt	24 pkt or 7¼ t	12 pkt or 4 t

Please keep in mind that aspartame must be added after cooking. We like to store our aspartame in little covered containers with a vanilla bean. We do this with Equal Measure® (the concentrated form) and NutraSweet Spoonful® (the measures-like-sugar type.)

We hope readers will find our dessert recipes helpful. If you are diabetic and also the cook, we hope our book will make your life easier. Why not just serve the same dessert to everyone in your family? You do not have to add an explanation. It's just chocolate cake or Grape-Nuts Pudding. For those of you readers who are not diabetic but are cooking for people who are, we hope these recipes will give you ideas on how to satisfy a sweet tooth safely. Although we clearly are not in charge of the other person's diabetes, we can do things that help. Cooking appropriate foods including desserts is one good way.

CHAPTER TWO

Cakes, Tortes, and Cake Rolls

Making "diabetic" cakes is a challenge; we offer you some tips here. Because sugar is needed to add lightness and a tender texture, it cannot be eliminated completely. We use a bare minimum of sugar and then bolster the sweet taste with artificial sweeteners. We substitute some new no-fat products, such as nonfat sour cream, yogurt, buttermilk, mayonnaise, cream cheese, etc. We offer a few other hints on making "diabetic" cakes.

* Watch cakes carefully near the end of the baking time. Low-sugar, low-fat cakes can easily overcook. Set your timer for the minimum time, then test for doneness. With most cakes, a toothpick inserted in the middle should come out clean.
* Use lots of beaten egg whites to add a light touch; using a minimum amount of sugar and fat can lead to a dense texture. You may want to save the unwanted egg yolks as "pet" food; animals don't suffer from cholesterol problems as some humans do.
* It often works well to use cake flour rather than regular flour. This too lightens a low-sugar, low-fat product.
* Bake cakes in fairly small containers to minimize the amount of time needed for baking. In larger pans cakes with only egg whites can become rubbery. Cupcake pans work well, as do small loaf pans.
* Slice leftover cake and freeze the individual slices well wrapped. That way you can defrost just the right amount. Do not expect low-sugar, low-fat cakes to remain fresh for a long time. Freezing works well. Take a few strawberries or raspberries out of a freezer bag and serve them with a defrosted cake slice.
* A person with a sweet tooth may want a little extra sweetness. As soon as a cake is out of the oven, poke a few holes in the top with a fork and drizzle in aspartame dissolved in an equal amount of water. Cupcakes can be rolled in the dissolved aspartame.

Making frosting is another real challenge since traditional frostings are basically mixtures of sugar and fat. The challenge is to make something that tastes good. A combination of artificial sweetener, cornstarch, and nonfat dry milk may look like frosting but the taste is disappointing. Our frosting recipes, based on ingredients such as nonfat cream cheese, are quite tasty. But to be honest, plan to serve the cake within a few hours of frosting it. These frostings do not have the staying power of sugary, fatty frostings. You can eliminate frosting by serving a slice of cake with a small amount of unsweetened applesauce; try adding a little cinnamon and aspartame. Or try our other Magic Touches from the appendix.

Our frosting recipes give the number of calories, exchanges, etc., per tablespoon. That way you can figure according to how many tablespoons (mL) you are eating.

Gingerbread

This cake looks ordinary, but the taste is quite special. If you want to add something on top, try our Lemon Sauce or an appropriate whipped topping.

1 C	flour	250 mL
¾ t	baking soda	4 mL
1 t	cinnamon	5 mL
½ t	dry mustard	2.5 mL
1 t	ginger	5 mL
dash	salt (optional)	dash
2 T	nonfat yogurt	30 mL
2 T	melted margarine or butter	30 mL
¼ C	molasses	40 mL
6 pkts	concentrated acesulfame-K	6 pkts
2 T	Prune Puree (page 138)	30 mL
3	egg whites	3

Glaze ingredients

2 T	hot water	30 mL
2 t	measures-like-sugar aspartame	10 mL
½ t	lemon extract	2.5 mL

Sift together the flour, baking soda, cinnamon, mustard, ginger, and salt. Set aside. In a separate bowl, whisk together the yogurt, margarine, molasses, acesulfame-K, and prune puree. Add the flour-and-spice mixture to the wet mixture and stir together. In a separate bowl, beat the egg whites until stiff. Gradually beat the beaten egg whites into the batter. Pour the batter into an 8-inch (20 cm) round pan that has been sprayed with non-stick vegetable cooking spray. Bake in a preheated 325°F (160°C) oven for 20–25 minutes or until a toothpick comes out clean. As soon as the gingerbread is out of the oven, combine the glaze ingredients. Use a toothpick to poke holes in the top of the gingerbread. Then use a pastry brush to brush the glaze over the top.

Yield: 10 servings **Exchange:** 1 bread
Each serving contains:
Calories: 89 Fiber: 0.4 g
Sodium: 130 mg Cholesterol: 0

Angel Food Cake I

Did you know that you should "break" angel food cake apart instead of using a knife to slice it? With a knife you compress the cake. Instead, use a special slicer or take two forks (one in each hand), and starting with the inside hole, jab the tines into the cake, keeping the forks very close together. Then work a line across to the outside by tearing the cake as you gently separate the forks.

1 C	flour	250 mL
¼ C	sugar	60 mL
3 pkts	concentrated acesulfame-K	3 pkts
1½ C	egg whites (12)	375 mL
1½ t	cream of tartar	7 mL
¼ t	salt	60 mL
¼ C	sugar	60 mL
4 pkts	concentrated acesulfame-K	4 pkts
1½ t	vanilla extract	7 mL
½ t	almond extract	2 mL

Sift together the flour, first amount of sugar, and first amount of acesulfame-K. Set aside. In a large mixing bowl, combine the egg whites, cream of tartar, and salt. With an electric mixer, beat until foamy. Mix together the second amount of sugar and the second acesulfame-K. Gradually add this mixture, a tablespoon (15 mL) at a time, to the egg whites. Continue beating until stiff peaks form. Fold in the vanilla and almond extracts. Sprinkle the flour mixture over the beaten egg whites. Fold gently just until the flour disappears. Fold the batter into an ungreased 10 × 4-inch (25 × 10 cm) tube pan.

Bake in a 375° (190°C) oven for 30–35 minutes, until no imprint remains after finger lightly touches the top of the cake. The top should be golden brown. To cool, turn the baked cake over. For best results stand the tube pan on a custard cup or put a bottle in the center hole to hold the top away from the counter so circulation will occur. Remove the cake from the pan only after it is thoroughly cool. Drizzle with bittersweet topping, fruit topping, or sliced fresh fruit.

Yield: 24 slices   **Exchange:** ½ bread
Each slice contains:
Calories: 42   Fiber: 1 g
Sodium: 178 mg   Cholesterol: 0.7 mg

Angel Food Cake II

During a recent insulin reaction, Edith's friend Bob wondered aloud why he had low blood sugar and thought it was because he had eaten some of this angel cake. Edith reminded him that the cake was only egg whites, flour and almost no sugar. The cake tastes so sweet, Bob had been fooled. And he hates artificial sweeteners.

¼ C	sugar	60 mL
½ C	measures-like-sugar saccharin	125 mL
6 pkts	concentrated acesulfame-K	6 pkts
1¼ C	cake flour	310 mL
12	egg whites	12
1½ t	cream of tartar	7 mL
pinch	salt (optional)	pinch
1 t	vanilla extract	5 mL
1 t	almond extract	5 mL

Stir together the sugar, measures-like-sugar saccharin, and acesulfame-K. Divide approximately in half. Set aside one half. Put the other half of the sugar-substitute/acesulfame-K mixture in a sifter with all the cake flour. Sift twice and set aside. Using an electric mixer, beat the egg whites with the cream of tartar, salt, and vanilla and almond extracts. Gradually add the reserved sugar-substitute/acesulfame-K mixture to the beaten egg whites. They should hold stiff peaks. Fold in the flour-sugar mixture, a small amount at a time, until it is all folded in.

Pour the batter into an angel cake pan that has been sprayed very lightly with non-stick cooking spray. Bake in a preheated 375°F (190°C) oven for 40 minutes or until the top is lightly browned, or until a toothpick inserted comes out clean. As soon as it is out of the oven, invert the pan on a rack and let cool completely before removing from the pan.

Yield: 24 servings   **Exchange:** ½ bread
Each serving contains:
Calories: 45   Fiber: 0
Sodium: 26 mg   Cholesterol: 0

Shortcake

People who like genuine shortcake with their strawberries or peaches will love this! Of course, others enjoy enjoy angel cake as a base for sweetened fruit. Those who wish to cut back on calories or exchanges can spoon fruit over half a shortcake.

1¾ C	flour	340 mL
1 t	sugar	5 mL
3 pkts	concentrated acesulfame-K	3 pkts
2 t	baking powder	10 mL
½ t	baking soda	1 mL
dash	salt (optional)	dash
3 T	margarine or butter	45 mL
⅝ C	nonfat milk or nonfat buttermilk	150 mL

Combine the flour, sugar, acesulfame-K, baking powder, baking soda, and salt. Cut in the margarine. Using a food processor makes this very quick and easy. Then add the milk and process, or use your hands to gather the dough into a ball.

Put the dough on a lightly floured surface. Work it briefly into a ball and then flatten it. Use a rolling pin to flatten it out; the dough should be about ¾-inch (1.75 cm) thick. Use a round biscuit cutter to cut out 10 circles. Place the biscuits on a baking sheet. Bake in a preheated 450°F (230°C) oven for 8–9 minutes, until lightly brown.

To serve, halve each biscuit and serve with fruit and whipped topping, if desired.

Yield: 10 servings   **Exchange:** 1 bread + ½ fat
     Each serving contains:
     Calories: 111   Fiber: trace
     Sodium: 103 mg   Cholesterol: trace

Hot-Milk Sponge Cake

This is one of Karin's grandmother's recipes updated with acesulfame-K. It uses fewer eggs than traditional sponge cake because the hot milk provides liquid.

1 C	sifted cake flour	250 mL
1 t	baking powder	5 mL
3	eggs	3
¼ C	sugar	60 mL
3 pkts	concentrated acesulfame-K	3 pkts
¼ C	hot milk	60 mL

1 t	vanilla extract	5 mL
	fruit (optional)	
	whipped topping (optional)	

Grease two 8-inch (30 cm) round layer-cake pans. Dust lightly with flour and baking powder mixed together. Using an electric mixer at high speed, beat the eggs in a small, deep bowl until they are light and fluffy; slowly beat in the sugar and acesulfame-K until the mixture is almost double in volume and is very thick. Turn the speed to low; beat in the hot milk and vanilla. Fold in the flour mixture, a third at a time, until just blended. Pour into the prepared pan.

Bake in a 350°F (180°C) oven for 15–20 minutes or until the centers spring back when lightly pressed with a fingertip. Cool in the pans on wire racks for 10 minutes. Then loosen cakes carefully around the edges with a knife, turn out onto the wire racks, and cool completely. To serve, put fresh fruit (or well-drained canned fruit packed in its own unsweetened juice) and your favorite whipped topping between the two layers and on top of the cake.

Yield: 8 servings **Exchange:** 1 bread
Each serving contains:
Calories: 108 Fiber: 0
Sodium: 79 mg Cholesterol: 103 mg

Oat Bran Cake

Oat bran is recommended especially for diabetics because it can help stabilize blood sugar. Here's a delicious way to serve it. Use the whole batter to make four large oat bran pancakes, about the size of a small cake. To turn this into a cake, assemble them in a stack with fillings in between. We like this combination.

1	pancake (recipe on page 139)	1
¼ C	raspberry or strawberry puree	60 mL
1	pancake	1
¼ C	Lemon Curd (see page 139) or	60 mL
1	pancake	1
¼ C	raspberry or strawberry puree	60 mL
1	pancake	1
¼ C	whipped topping	60 mL

Cut and serve like a cake.

Yield: 8 servings

Boston Cream Pie

No one will ever guess this is a diabetic dessert. Your guests will be impressed.

2 C	cake flour	500 mL
1 T	baking powder	15 mL
¼ t	salt (optional)	1 mL
1 C	egg substitute	250 mL
⅓ C	sugar	90 mL
6 pkts	concentrated saccharin	6 pkts
1½ t	vanilla extract	7 mL
½ t	butter-flavored extract	2 mL
⅓ C	canola oil	90 mL
1 C	egg whites at room temperature	250 mL
½ t	cream of tartar	2 mL

Cream Filling

1½ C	skim milk	375 mL
1 pkg.	fat-free, sugar-free vanilla instant pudding	1pkg.

Chocolate Topping

½	cream filling (above)	½
1 T	cocoa	15 mL

Sift together the flour, baking powder, and salt. Set aside. In a separate bowl, beat the egg substitute until light and fluffy. Add the sugar, saccharin, vanilla and butter extracts. Add the oil. Add the flour mixture. In another bowl, beat the egg whites until thick. Add the cream of tartar and continue beating until stiff. Stir about one-third of the stiff egg whites into the flour mixture to lighten. Then fold in the remaining egg whites. Pour into two 8-inch (20 cm) cake pans that have been coated with non-stick cooking spray. Bake in a preheated 350°F (180° C) oven for 25 minutes or until done.

To make the cream filling: Mix together the milk and pudding mix until thick. Spread half the cream filling between the layers.

To make the chocolate topping: Combine the other half of the cream topping with cocoa. Spread on top of the cream pie.

Yield: 12 servings   **Exchange:** 1 bread + 1 milk
        Each serving contains:
        Calories: 172   Fiber: 0.5 g
        Sodium: 63 mg   Cholesterol: 0.5 mg

Rich Chocolate Cake

Don't let the long list of ingredients intimidate you; this cake is worth the effort!

1⅓ C	cake flour	340 mL
⅓ C	unsweetened cocoa powder	90 mL
¼ t	baking powder	1 mL
¼ t	baking soda	1 mL
pinch	salt (optional)	pinch
½ C	egg substitute	125 mL
1 t	vanilla extract	5 mL
1 T	raspberry liqueur	45 mL
½ C	nonfat buttermilk	125 mL
4 T	margarine or butter	90 mL
2 T	prune puree	30 mL
15 pkts	concentrated acesulfame-K	15 pkts
3 T	sugar	45 mL
6	egg whites	6
¼ t	cream of tartar	1 mL
½ C	frozen raspberries	125 mL
½ t	concentrated aspartame	2 mL

Sift the first five ingredients together twice; set aside. Combine the egg substitute and vanilla extract, raspberry liqueur, and buttermilk. Using an electric mixer, cream the margarine or butter and the prune puree. Add acesulfame-K and sugar and beat well. Gradually add the egg substitute alternately with the flour mixture. Beat until well combined. Beat the egg whites until stiff. Add the cream of tartar and continue beating. Add a small amount of egg whites to the batter to lighten it. With a rubber spatula, fold in the remaining beaten whites. Pour into two 8-inch (20 cm) round cake pans that have been coated with non-stick cooking spray. Bake in a preheated 350°F (180°C) oven for 30–35 minutes. Cool, then invert onto a plate. Combine the raspberries and aspartame in a food processor to make raspberry puree. Spread raspberry puree over the top of one layer. Put the other layer on top and cover with raspberry puree.

Decorate top with whole raspberries if desired.

Yield: 10 servings   **Exchanges:** 2 bread + ½ fat
· **Each serving contains:**
Calories: 189   Fiber: 1.74 g
Sodium: 90 mg   Cholesterol: 0

Chocolate Tube Cake

Beaten egg whites make this cake rise high and give it a light texture. For a festive touch, put each slice on a decorative plate, add a dollop of whipped topping to each slice, and drizzle Bittersweet Sauce (page 147) over the top.

½ C	unsweetened cocoa powder	125 mL
¾ C	boiling water	190 mL
1¾ C	cake flour	440 mL
2 t	baking powder	10 mL
½ t	baking soda	2 mL
½ t	salt (optional)	2 mL
½ C	fructose	125 mL
½ C	egg substitute	125 mL
½ C	prune puree	125 mL
2 t	vanilla extract	2 mL
1 C	egg whites (room temperature)	250 mL
½ t	cream of tartar	2 mL

Pour the cocoa into boiling water and stir until smooth, then set aside to cool. Sift together the flour, baking powder, baking soda, salt, and fructose. In a bowl, beat the egg substitute, prune puree, and vanilla extract. Add the flour and cocoa mixtures to it and beat until smooth. In a separate bowl, beat the egg whites until foamy; add the cream of tartar, and continue beating until stiff. Stir about a third of the egg whites into the flour mixture to lighten it, then gently fold in the remaining whites. Pour the mixture into a tube pan coated with non-stick cooking spray. Bake in a preheated 325°F (160°C) oven for approximately an hour. The cake is done when it springs back when touched.

Yield: 12 servings   **Exchange:** 2 breads
Each serving contains:
Calories: 133   Fiber: 1.3 g
Sodium: 162 mg   Cholesterol: 0

Chocolate Eclair Cake

Karin made this for her mother's 75th-birthday party. It was easy to make, looked impressive, and tasted delicious. Everyone gave it rave reviews.

Dough

1 C	water	250 mL
½ C	canola oil	125 mL
1 C	flour	250 mL
4	eggs	4

1 t	butter-flavored extract	5 mL

Filling

2 (8 oz.) pkg	sugar-free vanilla pudding	2 (244 g) pkg
2½ C	skim milk	625 mL
¾ C	prepared sugar-free, low-fat whipped topping from mix	190 mL

Topping

6 T	unsweetened cocoa powder	90 mL
2 T	canola oil	30 mL
2 T	skim milk	30 mL
¾ C	aspartame	190 mL
1 t	vanilla extract	5 mL
	extra milk, if needed	
1 t	butter-flavored extract	5 mL

To make the dough: Heat the water and oil to a rolling boil. Stir in the flour over low heat until the mixture forms a ball. Remove from the heat. Using an electric mixer, beat in the eggs thoroughly, one at a time. Put in the butter extract. Spoon onto an ungreased cookie sheet in the shape of a ring or wreath. Bake until golden brown and dry at 400°F (200°C) for 35 to 40 minutes. Cool away from drafts. Slice in half horizontally. Just before serving add the filling by removing the top half, adding the filling, and replacing the top. Add the topping.

To make the filling: Whisk the pudding and milk until the mixture thickens. Fold in the whipped topping.

To make the topping: Melt the cocoa powder with the oil and milk. Cool. Add the aspartame and vanilla and beat until the mixture is the desired consistency. Add a little extra milk if necessary, one teaspoon at a time. Drizzle on top of the cake.

Yield: 24 servings   **Exchange:** 1 bread + 1 fat
Each serving contains:
Calories: 100   Fiber: trace
Sodium: 156 mg   Cholesterol: trace

Devil's Food Mayonnaise Cake

Fat-free mayonnaise works well to cut down on the calories, but you'd never guess this wasn't authentic devil's food.

2 t	baking soda	10 mL
1 C	cold water	250 mL
1 C	fat-free mayonnaise	250 mL
¼ C	unsweetened cocoa powder	60 mL
¼ C	sugar	60 mL
¼ C	measures-like-sugar saccharin	60 mL
2 C	flour	500 mL
1 t	vanilla extract	5 mL
2 C	whipped topping	500 mL

Dissolve the baking soda in water in a large mixing bowl. Stir in mayonnaise, cocoa, sugar and saccharin. Add flour, baking soda–water mixture, and vanilla and beat until smooth. Bake in two 8-inch (20 cm) cake pans at 350°F (180°C) for 30 to 35 minutes. Cool. Top with sugar-free whipped topping.

Yield: 10 servings   **Exchange:** 1½ bread
Each serving contains:
Calories: 132   Fiber: 0.5 g
Sodium: 479 mg   Cholesterol: 0

Applesauce-Carrot Cake

Carrot cakes tend to be very high in fat because of the large amount of oil used. This recipe gets its moist good taste from pineapple, applesauce, and nonfat sour cream. It has a wonderful texture and tastes very rich.

2 C	flour	500 mL
2 t	baking powder	10 mL
2 t	baking soda	10 mL
1 T	cinnamon	15 mL
1 t	allspice	5 mL
1 t	nutmeg	5 mL
½ C	pineapple, canned, crushed	125 mL
¼ C	raisins	60 mL
½ C	walnuts, chopped	125 mL
¼ C	sugar	60 mL
3 pkts	concentrated acesulfame-K	3 pkts
¾ C	egg substitute or 3 eggs	190 mL
½ C	measures-like-sugar saccharin	125 mL

½ C	nonfat sour cream	125 mL
½ C	unsweetened applesauce	125 mL
2 t	vanilla extract	10 mL
2 C	shredded carrots	500 mL
⅔ C	shredded coconut (optional)	180 mL

Sift together the flour, baking powder, baking soda, and spices. In a blender or food processor, blend the pineapple, raisins, nuts, and sugar. Do not liquefy. Mix together the acesulfame-K, eggs, saccharin, sour cream, applesauce, vanilla, and the blender mixture. Beat well. Add the flour mixture. Mix well. Add the carrots and coconut. Stir gently. Pour into a 10-inch (25 cm) cake pan coated with non-stick cooking spray. Bake at 350°F (180°C) for 50–60 minutes or until a cake tester inserted into the center comes out clean. Cool in the pan on a cooling rack. Remove from the pan and cut horizontally to make a two-layer cake. Frost between the layers and on top with Applesauce-Carrot Cake Frosting (recipe below).

Yield: 12 servings　　**Exchange:** 2 breads
Each serving contains:
Calories: 165　　Fiber: 1.6 g
Sodium: 304 mg　　Cholesterol: 1.3 mg

Applesauce-Carrot Cake Frosting

Although this is a variation of the classic carrot cake frosting, you might want to try it on other flavorful cakes as well.

8 oz.	nonfat cream cheese, softened	250 mL
½ C	bulk aspartame	125 mL
1 t	lemon extract	5 mL
1 t	butter-flavored extract	5 mL

Beat all ingredients together until smooth.

Yield: 12 T　　**Exchange:** free
1 T (15 mL) contains:
Calories: 17　　Fiber: 0
Sodium: 90 mg　　Cholesterol: 2.7 mg

Strawberry Layer Cake

This unusual recipe is adapted from a traditional Swedish dessert. Karin makes it for her family to top off a simple dinner.

3	eggs or equivalent egg substitute	3
¼ C	sugar	60 mL
3 pkts	concentrated acesulfame-K	3 pkts
1 C	flour	250 mL
2 t	baking powder	10 mL
8 T	margarine or butter, melted	125 mL
1 C	applesauce, unsweetened	250 mL
10 oz.	frozen strawberries, defrosted and unsweetened	300 g

Lightly oil a 6–8-inch (15–20 cm) skillet or griddle and heat it over low flame on the top of the stove. Beat the eggs, sugar, and acesulfame-K in a mixing bowl on high speed until they are thick. Sift together the flour and baking powder. Add the flour mixture to the egg mixture and mix gently by hand. Add the margarine and mix gently. Pour about ½ C (125 mL) of batter into the heated skillet; the batter should cover the bottom of the pan and be about the thickness of a pancake. Bake in a preheated 375°F (180°C) oven for 5 minutes, until the cake is lightly browned. Use a spatula to remove the layer to a serving plate. Pour another ½ C (125 mL) of batter into the skillet, and repeat. Blend the applesauce and strawberries together. Spread a layer of fruit between each of the three layers and on the top. Add your favorite whipped topping. Serve within six hours for best results.

Yield: 8 servings   **Exchange:** 1 bread + 2 fat
          Each serving contains:
          Calories: 162   Fiber: 1.3 g
          Sodium: 277 mg   Cholesterol: 0

Holiday Cranberry Cake

It's worth keeping cranberries in the freezer so you can make this cake year-round. Buy cranberries around Thanksgiving, when stores are well stocked with them.

2 C	cake flour	500 mL
1 t	baking powder	5 mL
½ t	baking soda	2 mL
pinch	salt (optional)	pinch
2 T	orange peel granules	30 mL
4 T	margarine or butter	60 mL

¼ C	sugar	30 mL
12 pkts	concentrated acesulfame-K	12 pkts
2 C	cranberries (fresh or frozen)	500 mL
½ C	egg substitute	125 mL
¾ C	nonfat sugar-free plain yogurt	190 mL
¼ C	Triple Sec	60 mL
1 t	vanilla extract	5 mL

Glaze

2 oz.	nonfat cream cheese	60 mL
1 t	concentrated aspartame	5 mL
2 T	skim milk	30 mL
½ t	clear vanilla extract	2 mL

Sift together the first four ingredients, add the orange peel, and set aside. With an electric mixer, soften the margarine. Add the sugar and acesulfame-K and beat for a few minutes. Add the egg substitute slowly and beat. Alternately add the flour mixture and the yogurt, liqueur, and vanilla extract. Beat for a few minutes, then fold in the cranberries. Pour the batter into a tube pan that has been coated with non-stick cooking spray. Bake in a preheated 350°F (180°C) oven for 45 minutes. Cool and then remove from the pan. Prepare the glaze and drizzle it over the top of the cake.

To make the glaze, soften the cream cheese by microwaving it for about 20 seconds or by heating it in a saucepan over very low heat. Set aside. Use a wire whisk to combine the other ingredients; then whisk in the softened cream cheese for a few minutes until it is creamy. Use large spoon to drizzle glaze over top of the cake.

Yield: 12 servings   **Exchange:** 1 fruit + 1 bread
Each serving contains:
Calories: 164   Fiber: 1 g
Sodium: 178 mg   Cholesterol: 0.7 mg

Apricot Loaf

Adding a glaze of dissolved aspartame gives this loaf a nice glossy look, as well as helping to satisfy a sweet tooth.

1 C	apricots	250 mL
2½ C	flour	625 mL
2 t	baking powder	10 mL
1 t	baking soda	5 mL
dash	salt (optional)	dash
2 T	grated orange rind	30 mL
¼ C	sugar	60 mL
9 pkts	concentrated acesulfame-K	9 pkts
2	egg whites	2
⅔ C	skim buttermilk	180 mL
⅔ C	orange juice	180 mL
1 t	vanilla extract	5 mL
¼ C	unsweetened applesauce	60 mL

Glaze ingredients

1 t	cornstarch	5 mL
¼ C	water	60 mL
2 t	measures-like-sugar aspartame	10 mL
½ t	orange extract	2.5 mL

Snip the apricots into small pieces with a pair of scissors. Set aside. Combine the flour, baking powder, baking soda, salt, orange rind, sugar, and acesulfame-K in a bowl. Add the apricot pieces and stir to combine. In a separate container, beat the egg whites and combine with the buttermilk, orange juice, vanilla extract, and applesauce. Add the wet ingredients to the dry ones, stirring until just combined. Do not overmix. Pour into a 9 × 5-inch (23 × 13 cm) loaf pan that has been sprayed with non-stick vegetable cooking spray. Bake in a preheated 350°F (180°C) oven for 50 minutes.

Prepare the glaze as follows. Combine the cornstarch and water in a small saucepan. Heat over medium heat; stir with a wire whisk until thickened. Turn off the heat, stir in the aspartame and extract. As soon as the bread is out of the oven, turn it onto a plate. Use a toothpick to poke holes in the top. Mix the glaze and pour it over the top.

Yield: 20 servings   **Exchange:** 1 bread
Each serving contains:
Calories: 83   Fiber: 0.8 g
Sodium: 52 mg   Cholesterol: 0

Tomato Soup Cake

This is a diabetic version of a Depression-era recipe, popular then because eggs were so expensive. It tastes even better refrigerated.

¼ C	sugar	60 mL
½ C	canola oil	125 mL
2 C	flour	500 mL
1 t	cinnamon	5 mL
1 t	nutmeg	5 mL
1 t	ground cloves	5 mL
1	baking soda	5 mL
1 t	baking powder	5 mL
¼ C	measures-like-sugar saccharin	60 mL
1 (10 oz.) can	tomato sauce	1 (300 g) can
1 C	raisins	250 mL

Frosting

1 (3 oz.) pkg	fat-free cream cheese	1 (90 g) pkg
1 C	measures-like-sugar aspartame	250 mL
1 t	vanilla extract	5 mL
1 T	evaporated skim milk	15 mL
1 t	butter-flavored extract	5 mL

Combine the sugar and oil in large bowl. Sift the dry ingredients together and add them to the sugar–oil mixture. Mix well. Add the soup and raisins. Turn into a loaf pan coated with non-stick cooking spray. Bake at 350°F (180°C) for 45 minutes. Cool. Frost with cream cheese frosting just before serving.

To make the frosting: With an electric mixer, whip the ingredients together.

Yield: 24 servings   **Exchange:** 1 bread + 1 fat + ½ milk
Each serving contains:
Calories: 143   Fiber: 4.5 g
Sodium: 795 mg   Cholesterol: trace

French Pastry Cake

The word for this cake is "Wow!" It would have been out of this world in fat and calories before the new nonfat ingredients, but once the cake is made, no one can tell.

½ C	margarine or butter	125 mL
½ C	nonfat cream cheese	125 mL
¼ C	sugar	60 mL
½ C	measures-like-sugar saccharin	125 mL
2	eggs or equivalent egg substitute	2
1 C	nonfat sour cream	250 mL
1 C	nonfat mayonnaise	250 mL
1 T	vanilla extract	15 mL
2 C	flour	500 mL
1 t	baking powder	5 mL
1 t	baking soda	5 mL

Cinnamon Mixture

1 T	cinnamon	15 mL
2 pkts	concentrated acesulfame-K	2 pkts
½ C	chopped almonds	½ C

Cream margarine or butter and cream cheese with sugar and saccharin. Add the eggs, sour cream, mayonnaise, and vanilla extract; beat well. Mix the flour, baking powder, and baking soda and add to the batter. Put half the batter into a tube pan or bundt pan coated with non-stick cooking spray. Mix together the cinnamon, acesulfame-K, and chopped almonds. Sprinkle half the cinnamon mixture on top of the batter in the pan, then add the rest of the batter. Sprinkle the rest of the cinnamon mixture on top of the batter. Bake at 350°F (180°C) 60–75 minutes or until the top is light brown and the cake pulls away from the pan.

Yield: 20 servings   **Exchange:** 1 fat + 1 bread
Each serving contains:
Calories: 155   Fiber: 0.6 g
Sodium: 274 mg   Cholesterol: 30 mg

Banana Tea Bread

This is great for occasions where a little something to go with coffee or tea is required.

½ C	egg substitute	125 mL
1 C	ripe banana, mashed	250 mL
1 t	vanilla extract	5 mL
2 C	flour	500 mL
½ t	salt (optional)	2 mL
1 t	baking soda	5 mL
2 T	sugar	30 mL
6 pkts	concentrated acesulfame-K	6 pkts

Glaze

2 T	boiling water	30 mL
4 t	concentrated aspartame	20 mL

Beat the egg substitute with a wire whisk; add the mashed banana and vanilla extract. Sift together the flour, salt, baking soda, sugar, and acesulfame-K. Add these dry ingredients to the egg-banana mixture and stir. Turn the mixture into a loaf pan that has been coated with non-stick cooking spray. Bake in a preheated 350°F (180°C) oven for 40 minutes.

After the bread is out of the oven, poke holes all over the top using a fork. Combine boiling water and aspartame; and use a pastry brush to cover top with glaze, letting the glaze sink into the holes.

Yield: 20 servings **Exchange:** 1 bread
Each serving contains:
Calories: 66 Fiber: 6 g
Sodium: 69 mg Cholesterol: 0

Banana Cake

Egg whites lighten this cake. You'll be proud to serve it.

2 C	flour	500 mL
1 T	baking powder	15 mL
2 T	fructose	30 mL
¼ C	fat-free mayonnaise	60 mL
½ C	egg substitute	125 mL
1½ C	mashed banana	375 mL
½ t	vanilla extract	2 mL
1 t	banana extract	5 mL
3	egg whites	3
¼ t	cream of tartar	1 mL

Sift together the flour, baking powder, and fructose. In a bowl, mix the mayonnaise, egg substitute, banana, and flavorings. Beat until smooth. Gradually add the flour mixture and beat to combine.

In a separate bowl, beat the egg whites until foamy. Add cream of tartar and beat until stiff. Add approximately a third of the whites to the flour mixture to lighten it. Gently fold in the rest.

Pour into two 8-inch (20 cm) cake pans that have been coated with nonstick cooking spray. Bake in a 350°F (180°C) oven for 20 minutes. Frost with Applesauce-Carrot Cake Frosting (page 23), Creamy Frosting (page 141), or your favorite whipped topping and sliced ripe bananas.

Yield: 12 servings   **Exchange:** 1½ bread
Each serving contains:
Calories: 121   Fiber: 1 g
Sodium: 183 mg   Cholesterol: 0

Macadamia Torte

This rivals fancy cakes in the best restaurants. No one would guess it's a diabetic recipe.

½ C	macadamia nuts, chopped fine	125 mL
¼ C	sugar	60 mL
1 C	measures-like-sugar saccharin	250 mL
1 t	baking soda	5 mL
2 C	flour	500 mL
1 t	baking powder	5 mL
1 t	ground ginger	5 mL
1	egg or equivalent egg substitute	1
⅔ C	canola oil	180 mL
1 C	nonfat sour cream	250 mL
1 t	vanilla extract	5 mL
1 t	butter-flavored extract	5 mL
¼ C	water	60 mL

Coat a 10-inch (25 cm) tube pan with non-stick cooking spray and sprinkle macadamia nuts evenly in the pan; set aside. Combine the dry ingredients in a large bowl. Combine the wet ingredients. Stir into the dry ingredients until smooth. Pour the batter into the prepared pan. Bake at 350°F (180°C) for 35 to 40 minutes or until a wooden pick inserted comes out clean. Cool 10 to 15 minutes.

Yield: 20 servings   **Exchange:** 1 bread + 2 fats
Each serving contains:
Calories: 153   Fiber: 0.6 g
Sodium: 99 mg   Cholesterol: 1.6 mg

Passover Chocolate-Nut Torte

This recipe contains no flour or leavening, so it is ideal for Passover—but it's worth making all year long.

½ C	walnut pieces, coarsely ground	125 mL
½ C	blanched almonds	125 mL
¼ C	sugar	60 mL
½ C	unsweetened cocoa powder	125 mL
3 pkts	concentrated acesulfame-K	3 pkts
1 T	cognac	15 mL
8	large egg whites	8

Put the nuts in a pie pan and bake in a 350°F (180°C) oven for about 10 minutes. Stir the nuts occasionally during toasting. Don't allow them to burn. Cool. Add sugar. Using a food processor, grind until powdery, but do not liquefy. Add the nuts and cocoa, acesulfame-K, and cognac. Pulse on and off until smooth and well combined. In a large bowl, beat the egg whites until stiff but not dry. Fold one quarter of the nut mixture into the egg whites and then fold that mixture into the rest of the nut mixture. Do not mix too much. Gently scrape into a 9-inch (23 cm) springform pan sprayed with non-stick cooking spray. Bake at 350°F (180°C) for 30 minutes. (A toothpick inserted into the center will *not* come out clean.) Cool on a wire rack before removing from the pan. Serve with your favorite whipped topping.

Yield: 12 servings   **Exchange:** ½ milk + 1 fat
Each serving contains:
Calories: 96   Fiber: 0.63 g
Sodium: 33 mg   Cholesterol: 0

Jelly Roll

As close to the bakery as you can get! To cut jelly-roll slices, slip a piece of 18-inch sewing thread under the roll. Crisscross the string on top of the jelly roll and pull quickly and evenly. Repeat for each slice.

1 C	sifted cake flour	250 mL
1 t	baking powder	5 mL
3	eggs	3
¼ C	sugar	60 mL
3 pkts	concentrated acesulfame-K	3 pkts
⅓ C	water	90 mL
1 t	vanilla extract	5 mL
¾ C	fruit-only raspberry, strawberry, or currant jelly	200 mL

Spray a 15 × 10 × 1-inch (37 × 25 × 3 cm) jelly-roll pan; line the bottom with wax paper; spray the paper. Sift the flour and baking powder together. With an electric mixer, beat the eggs in a medium bowl until thick and creamy and light in color. Gradually add the sugar and acesulfame-K, beating constantly until the mixture is very thick. Stir in the water and vanilla. Fold in the flour mixture. Spread the batter evenly in a prepared pan.

Bake at 375°F (190°C) for 12 minutes or until the center of the cake springs back when lightly pressed with a fingertip. Loosen the cake around the edges with a knife; invert the pan onto a clean tea towel; and peel off the wax paper. Starting at the short end, roll up the cake and towel together. Place the roll, seam-side down, on a wire rack and cool completely. When cool, unroll carefully. Spread evenly with jelly. To start rerolling, lift the end of the cake using the towel. Let the towel drop and, this time, just roll the cake. Place the roll, seam-side down, on a serving plate.

Yield: 20 slices   **Exchange:** 1 bread
Each serving contains:
Calories: 131   Fiber: 0
Sodium: 11 mg   Cholesterol: 48 mg

Fresh Strawberry Jelly Roll

Follow the jelly-roll recipe above. Cool the cake on a wire rack. Just before serving, unroll and spread with 1 C (250 mL) of your favorite sugar-free whipped topping and 1 C (250 mL) sliced strawberries. Reroll.

Mocha Chocolate Roll

There is only one word for this dessert: fabulous! *If we had to think of a second word, it would be "easy!"*

1 C	sifted cake flour	250 mL
¼ C	unsweetened cocoa powder	60 mL
1 t	baking powder	5 mL
3	eggs	3
¼ C	sugar	60 mL
3 pkts	concentrated acesulfame-K	3 pkts
⅓ C	cold coffee	90 mL
1 t	vanilla extract	5 mL

Filling

1 pkg	sugar-free whipped topping mix	1 pkg
½ C	cold, very strong coffee	125 mL

Spray a 15 × 10 × 1-inch (37 × 25 × 3 cm) jelly-roll pan; line the bottom with wax paper; spray the paper. Sift the flour, cocoa, and baking powder together. With an electric mixer, beat the eggs in a medium bowl until thick and creamy and light in color. Gradually add the sugar and acesulfame-K, beating constantly until the mixture is very thick. Stir in the coffee and vanilla extract. Fold in the flour mixture. Spread the batter evenly in a prepared pan.

Bake in a 350°F (180°C) oven for 12 minutes or until the center springs back when pressed lightly with a fingertip. Loosen the cake around the edges with a knife; invert the pan onto a clean tea towel. Peel off the wax paper. Starting at the short end, roll up the cake and towel together. Place the roll, seam-side down, on a wire rack; cool completely.

To make the filling, follow the directions for the whipped topping mix on the package but use cold coffee instead of water. When the cake is cool, unroll it carefully. Spread it evenly with filling. To start rerolling, lift the cake with the end of the towel. Place it, seam-side down, on a serving plate.

Yield: 20 servings   **Exchange:** ½ bread + ½ fat
Each serving contains:
Calories: 70   Fiber: 0
Sodium: 53 mg   Cholesterol: 41 mg

Spicy Prune Roll

A delightful jelly roll, very easy to make, with a great flavor.

¾ C	sifted cake flour	180 mL
1 t	baking powder	5 mL
½ t	ground cinnamon	2 mL
4	eggs	4
2 T	sugar	30 mL
3 pkts	concentrated acesulfame-K	3 pkts
1 t	vanilla extract	5 mL

Prune Filling

1 C	pitted prunes	250 mL
½ C	water or apple juice (unsweetened)	125 mL
½ T	lemon juice	7 mL
¼ t	ground cinnamon	1 mL

Grease a 15 × 10 × 1-inch (37 × 25 × 3 cm) jelly-roll pan; line it with wax paper; grease the paper. Measure the flour, baking powder, and cinnamon into a sifter. Beat the eggs in a medium bowl until foamy; gradually beat in the sugar and acesulfame-K until the mixture is very thick and light. Stir in the vanilla.

Sift the dry ingredients over the egg mixture; gently fold in until no streaks of flour remain. Spread the batter evenly in a prepared pan. Bake in a 375°F (190° C) oven for 12 minutes or until the center springs back when lightly pressed with a fingertip.

Loosen the cake around the edges with a knife; invert the pan onto a clean tea towel. Peel off the wax paper. Starting at the short end, roll up the cake and towel together. Place the roll, seam-side down, on wire rack. Cool completely.

Combine the prunes and water or apple juice in a small saucepan; simmer, covered, for 25 minutes. Puree the prunes with the remaining cooking liquid, part at a time, in a blender or food processor. Stir in the lemon juice and cinnamon. Chill.

When cake is cool, unroll it carefully. Spread it with filling. To start rerolling, lift the end of the cake with a towel. Place the roll, seam-side down, on a serving plate.

Yield: 20 slices   **Exchange:** 1 bread
    Each slice contains:
    Calories: 62   Fiber: 1 g
    Sodium: 34 mg   Cholesterol: 55 mg

Squash or Pumpkin Roll

A variation on the traditional jelly roll, this one has a cream-cheese filling and a lovely, moist cake.

3	eggs	3
¼ C	sugar	125 mL
3 pkts	concentrated acesulfame-K	3 pkts
1 t	lemon juice	5 mL
¾ C	canned squash or pumpkin	190 mL
¾ C	flour	190 mL
1 t	baking powder	5 mL
1 t	ginger	5 mL
2 t	cinnamon	10 mL
½ t	nutmeg	2 mL
1 C	chopped walnuts	250 mL

Filling

6 oz.	nonfat cream cheese	185 mL
4 T	margarine or butter	60 mL
½ t	butter-flavored extract	2 mL
½ t	vanilla extract	2 mL
2 T	sugar	30 mL
4 pkts	concentrated acesulfame-K	4 pkts

Beat eggs at high speed for 5 minutes until they are thick and light in color. Gradually add sugar, acesulfame-K, lemon, and squash. Sift the flour, baking powder, and spices all together and fold into the mixture. Mix well. Spread into a 10-inch (25 cm) jelly-roll pan lined with wax paper coated well with non-stick cooking spray. Spread nuts over the top. Bake at 375°F (190°C) for 12 minutes, until a toothpick inserted comes out clean. Turn onto a dish towel. Roll up with the towel in between. Cool.

To make the filling, whip together the cream cheese, margarine, and butter and vanilla extracts. Slowly add the sugar and acesulfame-K. Unroll the cake. Spread filling over the entire cake. Reroll and chill.

Yield: 20 slices   **Exchange:** ½ bread + 1 fat
Each slice contains:
Calories: 111   Fiber: 0.88 g
Sodium: 98 mg   Cholesterol: 42 mg

CHAPTER THREE

Cheesecakes

An entire chapter on cheesecakes! Why? Because the new nonfat dairy products make it easy to make cheescakes that fit into diabetic meal plans. These products also add calcium and protein. Here are a few hints about using these new nonfat products.

Nonfat ricotta cheese

Check the dates on the label before you buy; use the cheese while it's still fresh. Nonfat ricotta is used not only in cooking, it also makes a nice (and fat-free) spread for toast and other foods; try it with a little added nutmeg and aspartame.

Nonfat cottage cheese

Process in a food processor or blender for a full two to three minutes to eliminate the curds before using in cooking.

Nonfat cream cheese

Microwave for 30 seconds to soften before adding it to a recipe.

Yogurt

Don't be misled by clever labels. Be sure the yogurt is 100% nonfat. It should also be free of sugar and other caloric sweeteners such as fruit purees. Some yogurts are sweetened with only aspartame or NutraSweet.

Skim milk

Skim milk does not create rich, creamy desserts the way cream does, although it's fairly innocuous. So add a little cornstarch dissolved in water to thicken dishes made with skim milk. Opinions vary on the use of canned evaporated skim milk. Some people like it when it is disguised by tasty ingredients. One friend, however, refers to it as the kiss of death to any recipe's chances of tasting good.

Egg substitutes

These are a popular way to avoid cholesterol and are more convenient to use in cooking than whole eggs. Egg substitutes can be found in supermarkets either chilled near the eggs or frozen in the freezer section. Some egg substitutes are totally non-fat, others have a very small amount of fat. We had more success cooking with a defrosted egg substitute that has a tiny amount of corn oil than with the totally fat-free versions.

Egg substitutes and egg whites, which is basically what egg substitutes are, have a tendency to become rubbery, especially if exposed to too much heat. To minimize this problem, cook cheesecakes in a hot-water bath, the traditional way to bake custards. In a hot-water bath, food cooks in a smaller pan or pans set inside a larger pan of hot water.

Here's an easy way to manage: Preheat the oven, open the oven door, and slide the lower oven rack partway out. Set the larger pan on this rack. Put the smaller pan(s) of uncooked food in the center of the larger pan. Take a teakettle of boiling water and very carefully pour boiling water into the larger pan. Be sure you do not spill or splatter any water inside the smaller pan. Also, if you're using a springform pan, which is great for cheesecake, be sure the rim is tightly attached to the bottom rim.

Gelatin in cheesecake

Opinions vary on this subject. Some people declare vehemently that "real" cheesecake does not have gelatin. Others like gelatin-based desserts. We give you lots of choice; you decide which you prefer.

Crust

As far as crusts are concerned, you can decide for yourself. Some people like a graham cracker crust, which is described in the chapter on pies. To save calories, many cheesecake recipes suggest you simply sprinkle a few tablespoons of graham cracker crumbs on the base of the pan. Of course, you can make a cheesecake with no crust or bottom layer.

Granola Cheesecake

A super combination—creamy cheesecake with a crunch.

Crust

¼ C	margarine or butter, melted	60 mL
1 T	water	15 mL
3 pkts	concentrated acesulfame-K	3 pkts
1 C	Granola Topping, page 144	250 mL

Filling

8 oz.	nonfat cream cheese, softened	250 mL
1 C	nonfat cottage cheese, drained	250 mL
½ C	egg substitute or 2 eggs	125 mL
3 pkts	concentrated acesulfame-K	3 pkts
1 t	vanilla extract	5 mL
1 T	flour	15 mL

Topping

⅓ C	Granola Topping (see page 144)	90 mL

Stir the crust ingredients together and press the mixture into the bottom of a 9-inch (23 cm) springform pan. Set aside. Beat the filling ingredients together until smooth. Spoon this carefully over the crust. Sprinkle the top with granola topping. Bake in a 375°F (190°C) oven for 40 minutes or until set. Cool before removing cake from the pan.

Yield: 10 servings   **Exchange:** 1 meat
Each serving contains:
Calories: 88   Fiber: trace
Sodium: 186 mg   Cholesterol: 5.2 mg

Healthy Cheesecake

This is a healthy version of the old-fashioned cheesecake everyone loves. We don't think you'll miss the fat!

¼ C	graham cracker crumbs	60 mL
2 C	yogurt cheese*	500 mL
2 t	vanilla extract	10 mL
½ C	egg substitute	125 mL
2 T	cornstarch	30 mL
6 pkts	concentrated acesulfame-K	6 pkts

Topping

½ C	nonfat sour cream	125 mL
2 t	sugar	10 mL
2 t	concentrated acesulfame-K	2 t
1 t	vanilla extract	5 mL

Spray a 9-inch (23 cm) springform (or other) pie pan with non-stick cooking spray. Sprinkle it evenly with graham-cracker crumbs. Set aside.

Use an electric mixer to combine the next five ingredients. Beat until creamy. Pour the mixture onto the crumbs. Bake in a preheated 325°F (160°C) oven for 35 minutes. Remove from the oven and let cool. Refrigerate. Combine the topping ingredients and pour the mixture over the baked, chilled cheesecake. Return it to the oven for 10 minutes. Chill. Run a knife around the edge of the pan to loosen the cheesecake.

Yield: 12 servings   **Exchange:** ½ bread
Each serving contains:
Calories: 49   Fiber: trace
Sodium: 68 mg   Cholesterol: 2 mg

*Yogurt cheese is made by letting yogurt drip through cheesecloth overnight in the refrigerator.

Apple Cheesecake

This cheesecake is fabulous. Some people like to pour the batter into a pre-baked graham cracker crust.

1 lb.	nonfat cottage cheese	450 g
⅔ C	nonfat sour cream	180 mL
4 t	fructose	20 mL
2	eggs	2
1 T	all-purpose flour	15 mL
½ t	nutmeg	5 mL
pinch	cinnamon	pinch
1	juice of one lemon	1
4	small apples, peeled, cored, and sliced into half moons	4
	Graham-Cracker Crust (page 73)	(optional)

Beat the cottage cheese, sour cream, fructose, eggs, flour, nutmeg, and cinnamon until smooth. Stir in the lemon juice. Spread half the apples in the bottom, over a crust if you like. Pour the cottage cheese mixture over the apples. Top with the remaining apples. Bake in a preheated oven at 375°F (190°C) or until set. Cool completely.

Yield: 10 servings   **Exchange:** 1 bread
Each serving contains:
Calories: 101   Fiber: 1.1 g
Sodium: 36 mg   Cholesterol: 61 mg

Cheesecake with Jelly Glaze

This looks more like a pie than a cheesecake, but it tastes like a cheesecake. The top looks lovely with slices of kiwi and raspberry or strawberry halves.

1 (8 oz.) pkg	nonfat cream cheese	1 (250 mL) pkg
1 C	nonfat yogurt sweetened with aspartame	250 mL
1 pkg	unsweetened gelatin	1 pkg.
¼ C	water	90 mL
1 T	measures-like-sugar aspartame	15 mL
1 C	cut into pieces, fresh fruit, or canned, no sugar added	250 mL
3 T	jelly, made with saccharin	45 mL

Combine the cream cheese and yogurt and beat until smooth. In a small saucepan, sprinkle the gelatin into the water; let soften for 2 minutes. Over low heat, stir to dissolve the gelatin. Remove from the heat and add to cream cheese mixture. Add the aspartame. With an electric mixer, beat until smooth. Pour into a crust of your choice (A graham-cracker crust is traditional.) Arrange the fruit on top. Microwave the jelly for 30 seconds or heat in a saucepan over low heat. When jelly is liquefied, use a pastry brush to glaze the top of the pie.

Yield: 8 servings   **Exchange:** 1 milk
Each serving contains:
Calories: 60   Fiber: 0.5 g
Sodium: 164 mg   Cholesterol: 4 mg

Pumpkin Cheesecake

This is a wonderful cheesecake, creamy and smooth, with a hint of your favorite pumpkin-pie taste.

1 lb.	nonfat cream cheese	450 g
12 t	fructose	60 mL
¼ C	egg substitute	60 mL
1 (16 oz.) can	pumpkin	1 (488 mL) can
1½ t	cinnamon	7.5 mL
1 t	allspice	5 mL
¼ t	ginger	1.25 mL
¼ t	mace	1.25 mL
1	unbaked crust, preferably graham (optional)	1

Spray an 8-inch (20 cm) springform pan with non-stick vegetable cooking spray. Line the bottom of the sprayed pan with crust, if desired. Beat the cream cheese, fructose, and egg substitute until smooth. Beat the pumpkin and spices into the cheese mixture. Spoon the filling into the crust, if used. Bake in a preheated 350°F (180°C) oven for 45 minutes or until set. Cool the cake completely before removing it from the pan.

Yield: 10 servings   **Exchange:** 1 milk
Each serving contains:
Calories: 82   Fiber: 2 g
Sodium: 244 mg   Cholesterol: 6.4 mg

Ricotta Pie

This is a traditional Italian Easter dessert. You'll like it at any time of the year.

2 lb.	fat-free ricotta	900 g
6	eggs	6
⅓ C	sugar	90 mL
⅓ C	measures-like-sugar saccharin	90 mL
2 t	vanilla extract	10 mL
2 t	butter-flavored extract	10 mL
1 t	cinnamon	5 mL

With an electric mixer, beat all the ingredients except the cinnamon until smooth. Pour the batter into a 10-inch (25 cm) pie crust of your choice. Sprinkle with cinnamon. Bake at 350°F (180°C) for 50 to 60 minutes until a knife inserted comes out clean. Cool. Refrigerate.

Yield: 8 servings **Exchange:** 1½ milk + 1 meat
Each serving contains:
Calories: 159   Fiber: 1 g
Sodium: 178 mg   Cholesterol: 10 mg

No-Bake Orange Cheesecake

Make this a day or two ahead of time . Keep it covered and refrigerated until serving time. Garnish with the oranges just before serving.

Crust

1 C	finely crushed graham cracker crumbs	250 mL
3 T	melted margarine or butter	45 mL

Cheesecake Filling

¼ C	cold water	60 mL
1 env.	unflavored gelatin	1 env.
16 oz.	nonfat cream cheese, at room temperature	450 g
¼ C	sugar	60 mL
6 pkts	concentrated acesulfame-K	6 pkts
1 C	nonfat sour cream	250 mL
¾ C	freshly squeezed orange juice	180 mL
1 t	freshly grated orange peel	5 mL
2 t	orange flavoring	10 mL

Topping

3	navel oranges, peeled, bitter parts removed	3

To make the crust: Mix the graham-cracker crumbs and margarine. Spread this over the bottom and a little up the sides of a 9-inch (23 cm) springform pan. Freeze the crust while mixing the filling.

To make the filling: Put the water in a small saucepan and sprinkle the gelatin on top. After 1 minute turn the heat on low and, stirring constantly, heat for 2–3 minutes until the gelatin is dissolved. Remove from heat.

With an electric mixer, beat the cream cheese, sugar, and acesulfame-K in a large bowl. When the mixture is fluffy, add the sour cream and beat well. Mix in the orange juice, gelatin, peel, and flavoring. Pour into a chilled crust. Refrigerate for 4–6 hours until firm.

Before serving, run a thin knife around the edge of the cake to loosen it. Remove the springform from the outside. Top the cake with sliced oranges.

Yield: 12 servings   **Exchange:** 1 bread + ½ fat + ½ milk
Each serving contains:
Calories: 164   Fiber: 1.2 g
Sodium: 265 mg   Cholesterol: 9.1 mg

Creamy Amaretto Cheesecake

Our taste testers loved this almond-flavored cheesecake

2 (8 oz.) pkgs	nonfat cream cheese	2 (244 g) pkgs
2 T	cornstarch	30 mL
2 t	concentrated acesulfame-K	10 mL
2 T	sugar	30 mL
¼ C	Amaretto	60 mL
1 t	vanilla extract	5 mL
½ C	egg substitute	125 mL
1	graham cracker crust (optional)	1
	fresh fruit (optional)	

Cream the first six ingredients together. Pour in the egg substitute and beat with an electric mixer until creamy. Pour the batter into an 8-inch (20 cm) graham cracker crust, if desired. Bake in a preheated 325°F (160°C) oven for 35 minutes. Chill. Before serving, top with fruit, if desired.

Yield: 8 servings   **Exchange:** 1 milk
Each serving (without crust) contains:
Calories: 108   Fiber: 0
Sodium: 303 mg   Cholesterol: 8 mg

Strawberry Cream Cheese Tarts

These are very light and fluffy and have a wonderful, rich flavor. No one will guess they aren't loaded with fat and calories.

6 oz.	nonfat cream cheese	200 g
¾ C	nonfat cottage cheese	190 mL
⅔ C	nonfat sour cream	180 mL
3	eggs separated	3
7 t	fructose	35 mL
1	graham cracker crust recipe pressed into 18 tart pans	1

To prepare the filling, beat the cream cheese, cottage cheese, sour cream, egg yolks, and fructose in a large bowl until smooth. In another bowl, beat the egg whites until soft peaks form; fold them into the cheese mixture. Spoon the filling into the prepared crusts. Chill until set. Garnish with Strawberry Topping, page 145.

Yield: 18 tarts **Exchange:** ½ milk
Each tart contains:
Calories: 44 Fiber: 0
Sodium: 63 mg Cholesterol: 49 mg

Marble Cheesecake

This is a spectacular-looking dessert. We made it with 2 T (30 mL) sugar and remade it with fructose. Although the sugar version won out in the taste and texture contest, the fructose version was quite good too.

2 C	nonfat ricotta cheese	500 mL
8 oz.	nonfat cream cheese	250 g
¼ C	egg substitute	60 mL
3	egg whites	3
2 T	sugar	30 mL
12 pkts	concentrated acesulfame-K	12 pkts
1 T	vanilla extract	15 mL
1½ t	lemon juice	7.5 mL
3 T	cocoa	45 mL
3 T	water	45 mL
2 pkts	concentrated acesulfame-K	2 pkts
3 T	crumbs made from 2 chocolate cookies sweetened with fructose	45 mL

Put the ricotta cheese in a food processor or blender and process for a full minute. Soften the cream cheese in a microwave oven for 30 seconds. Add it to the food processor with the egg substitute, egg whites, sugar, acesulfame-K, vanilla extract, and lemon juice. Process to combine. In a medium bowl, whisk together the cocoa, water, and acesulfame-K.

Pour approximately 1 C (250 mL) cheese batter from the food processor into the cocoa. Whisk to combine. Set aside this "chocolate" batter. Then take a 9-inch (23 cm) springform baking pan that has been sprayed with non-stick vegetable cooking spray. Pour most of the white batter into this prepared pan. Pour all the chocolate batter in the center on top of the white batter. There will be a white ring all around the edge of the pan. Carefully pour the rest of the white batter into the center of the chocolate batter. Use a knife to marble the batters by making an "S" curve through the batter. Do not mix completely.

Place the springform pan in the center of a baking pan. Slowly and carefully pour boiling water into the outer baking pan, smoothing the batter in the springform pan. (This hot-water bath will help the cheesecake bake like a custard.) Bake in a preheated 325°F (160°C) oven for 50 minutes or until it starts to shrink away from the sides of the pan. Remove the cake from the hot-water bath and chill it completely overnight. Press chocolate cookie crumbs onto the sides of the cake.

Yield: 16 servings   **Exchange:** ½ milk
Each serving contains:
Calories: 57   Fiber: trace
Sodium: 112 mg   Cholesterol: 4.5 mg

Cheese Flan

You'll love serving this elegant dessert. It rivals the desserts in fancy restaurants, yet it's easy to make and virtually foolproof.

4	eggs or equivalent egg substitute	4
½ C	nonfat sour cream	125 mL
8 oz.	nonfat cream cheese	250 g
¼ C	lemon juice	125 mL
2 t	vanilla extract	10 mL
1 pkt	concentrated acesulfame-K	1 pkt
dash	nutmeg	dash
4 T	chopped walnuts	60 mL
2 T	measures-like-sugar aspartame	30 mL
1	unbaked crust (optional)	1

Spread the crust on the bottom of a flan pan or quiche dish. Put the next seven ingredients into a blender. Pour the blender contents onto a graham cracker or other crust, if desired. Bake at 375°F (190°C) for 25 minutes. Mix together the walnuts and aspartame. Sprinkle over the flan. Cool. Store the flan in the refrigerator.

Yield: 16 servings   **Exchange:** ½ milk
Each serving contains:
Calories: 41   Fiber: trace
Sodium: 111 mg   Cholesterol: 3 mg

CHAPTER FOUR

Cookies, Squares, and Other Finger Foods

Cookies present an inherent challenge in diabetic cooking. Without fat, cookies don't hold together. Without sugar, cookies don't have a nice light texture, don't rise up, and don't brown nicely. We present a collection of excellent cookie recipes with a minimum of sugar and the balance of sweetening added with artificial sweeteners .

Our best hint for serving cookies is to count out the appropriate number and then serve them on a small, decorative plate. When the cookies are presented, make it look like a special occasion. Serve tea from a pretty teapot in pretty teacups. Or serve the cookies with a cup of coffee, dietetic hot chocolate, or a glass of skim milk. Again, make snack time special by using nice napkins and place mats. For many people this helps satisfy a need to feel nurtured and loved.

Did you ever just stand up in the kitchen and munch cookies as you leaned against the counter? We've probably all done this when we were hungry or otherwise needy. It's all too easy to take in many too many calories and exchanges this way. So serve your cookies or squares or scones on a decorative plate and enjoy.

For some classic recipes, we offer a choice, because some people like their brownies rich and fudgy while others prefer cakelike ones.

No-Bake Coconut Surprise

An easy treat to whip together and store in the refrigerator.

1 (8 oz.) pkg.	nonfat cream cheese	1 (250 mL) pkg
1 pkt	concentrated acesulfame-K	1 pkt
1 T	walnuts, chopped	15 mL
1 t	orange extract	5 mL
¼ C	toasted flaked coconut	60 mL

Beat the cheese with acesulfame-K until light and fluffy; add the walnuts and the extract. Shape into 20 balls, each about ½ t. Roll each in coconut. Chill.

Yield: 20 cookies   **Exchange:** ½ meat
Each cookie contains:
Calories: 33   Fiber: trace
Sodium: 54 mg   Cholesterol: 1.6 mg

Cookie Cutter Cookies

Children and adults love cookies cut into shapes. If you like sprinkles, try dusting these with Crystal Light as they come out of the oven.

1 C	margarine or butter	350 mL
¼ C	sugar	60 mL
6 pkts	concentrated acesulfame-K	6 pkts
2½ C	flour	625 mL
1 t	baking soda	5 mL
1 t	cream of tartar	5 mL
1 t	vanilla extract	5 mL
1 t	almond extract	5 mL
1	egg or equivalent egg substitute	1

Cream the margarine and sugar. Stir in the rest of the ingredients one at a time in the order listed. Form the dough into a ball, wrap it in plastic wrap, and refrigerate it for at least two hours. Cut the dough into thirds. Roll each third ⅛-inch (5 mm) thick on a lightly floured board. Cut the dough into shapes with the cookie cutters. Place the cookies onto ungreased cookie sheets. Bake at 400°F (200°C) for 5–8 minutes.

Yield: 100 small cookies   **Exchange:** ½ fat
Each cookie contains:
Calories: 29   Fiber: trace
Sodium: 13 mg   Cholesterol: 0

Scones

Scones are wonderful with a cup of tea or coffee. These low-fat scones are best served the same day they're baked. So they're perfect for a special brunch or meeting over coffee.

2 C	flour	500 mL
1½ t	baking powder	7 mL
1½ t	baking soda	7 mL
dash	salt (optional)	dash
1½ T	sugar	22 mL
3 pkts	concentrated acesulfame-K	3 pkts
2 t	cinnamon	10 mL
3 T	margarine or butter	45 mL
⅔ C	nonfat yogurt, no sugar added	180 mL
2	egg whites	2

Combine in the bowl of a food processor the flour, baking powder, baking soda, salt, acesulfame-K, and cinnamon. Add the margarine cut into small pieces. Pulse the food processor off and on just long enough to combine; do not over-process. Add the yogurt and egg whites. Process very briefly. Turn this sticky dough out onto a lightly floured surface. Pat it out. Use a rolling pin to make a circle about ¾ inch (1.75 cm) thick and about 8 inches (20 cm) round. Cut into wedges as follows: Cut the circle in quarters, then cut each quarter into three sections. Place on a cookie sheet and bake in a pre-heated 425°F (220°C) oven for 15 minutes.

Yield: 12 scones   **Exchange:** 1 bread
Each scone contains:
Calories: 110   Fiber: trace
Sodium: 215 mg   Cholesterol: 0

Cinnamon Crescents

These cookies look very fancy when they are made up. They are yummy too!

1 C	margarine or butter	250 mL
2 C	flour, sifted	500 mL
1	egg yolk	1
¾ C	nonfat sour cream	190 mL
3 T	sugar	45 mL
3 pkts	concentrated acesulfame-K	3 pkts
¾ C	finely chopped walnuts	190 mL
2 t	cinnamon	10 mL
1	egg white, slightly beaten in 1 T (15 mL) water	1

Cut the margarine into the flour until the mixture resembles coarse crumbs. Stir in the egg yolk and sour cream. Form a ball. Cover with plastic wrap and chill for two hours. Combine the sugar, acesulfame-K, walnuts, and cinnamon. Divide the dough into fourths. Roll each into an 11-inch (28 cm) circle. Sprinkle with a quarter of the sugar mixture. Cut into 16 wedges. Roll up the wedges, starting at the widest end. Place the rolls on an ungreased cookie sheet. Brush with egg white and water. Bake in a 350°F (180°C) oven for 20 minutes or until golden brown. Cool on wire racks.

Yield: 48 cookies   **Exchange:** ½ bread + ½ fat
Each cookie contains:
Calories: 70   Fiber: trace
Sodium: 6.6 mg   Cholesterol: 6.2 mg

Snickerdoodles

New research has indicated that the smell of cinnamon baking is an aphrodisiac! These cookies may be the way to his (or her) heart.

1 C	margarine or butter	250 mL
¼ C	sugar	60 mL
6 pkts	concentrated acesulfame-K	6 pkts
2	eggs	2
1 t	vanilla extract	5 mL
2⅔ C	flour, sifted	690 mL
2 t	cream of tartar	10 mL
1 t	baking soda	5 mL

Coating

2 T	sugar	30 mL
1 t	cinnamon	5 mL

Beat the margarine until light. Add the sugar and acesulfame-K and beat until fluffy. Beat in the eggs and vanilla. Sift together the flour, cream of tartar, and baking soda. Add this to the margarine mixture.

Combine the sugar and cinnamon in a separate bowl. With floured hands, shape the dough into small balls about 1 inch (2.5 cm) apiece and roll each one in the sugar-cinnamon mixture. Place each 2 inches (5 cm) apart on an ungreased baking sheet. Bake at 400°F (200°C) for 8–10 minutes. Cool on wire racks.

Yield: 6 dozen cookies **Exchange:** ½ fat
Each cookie contains:
Calories: 44   Fiber: trace
Sodium: 18 mg   Cholesterol: 7.6 mg

Swedish Ginger Snaps

Karin's father used to roll out these cookies between waxed paper to get them very, very thin. They are called "pepparkakor" in Swedish, and for Christmas are cut into hearts, stars, and other Christmas shapes.

⅓ C	molasses	90 mL
1 t	ginger	5 mL
1 t	cinnamon	5 mL
½ t	ground cloves	2 mL
6 pkts	concentrated acesulfame-K	6 pkts
¾ T	baking soda	3 mL
⅔ C	margarine or butter	180 mL

⅔ C	nonfat sour cream	180 mL
¼ C	egg substitute (or 1 egg)	60 mL
5 C	sifted flour	1.25 L

In a saucepan, bring the molasses and spices to a boil. Remove from the heat and add the acesulfame-K, baking soda, and margarine. Stir until the margarine melts. Add the sour cream, egg substitute, and flour and mix thoroughly. Turn out onto lightly floured board and knead into a ball. Wrap in plastic wrap and refrigerate two hours or more. Roll a manageable amount of dough on a lightly floured board to a thickness of ¼-inch (55 mm) and cut with cookie cutters. Place on a cookie sheet coated with non-stick cooking spray. Bake at 325°F (160°C) for 8–10 minutes.

Yield: 250 very thin cookies   **Exchange:** free
Each cookie contains:
| Calories: 13 | Fiber: trace |
| Sodium: 12 mg | Cholesterol: trace |

Ruth's Dream Cookies

Ruth loved these cookies better than any we ever made.

½ C	margarine or butter	125 mL
¼ C	sugar	60 mL
6 pkts	concentrated acesulfame-K	6 pkts
½ C	nonfat cream cheese	125 mL
2 t	vanilla extract	10 mL
1 t	baking powder	5 mL
2 C	flour, sifted	500 mL
20	blanched almonds, halved	20

Brown the margarine slightly in a frying pan. Let it cool and transfer it to a bowl. Add the sugar, acesulfame-K, and cream cheese. Beat until smooth and blended. Add the vanilla and baking powder. Mix well. Add the flour and mix. The dough will be crumbly. Using your hands, roll the dough into smooth balls about the size of walnuts. Place each on a cookie sheet sprayed with non-stick cooking spray. Put half an almond on the top of each ball. Bake in a 250°F (120°C) oven until golden brown, about half an hour.

Yield: 40 cookies   **Exchange:** ½ bread + ½ fat
Each cookie contains:
| Calories: 51 | Fiber: trace |
| Sodium: 12 mg | Cholesterol: trace |

Amaretto Dreams

These fragile cookies are much like the ones that come in fancy packages at the grocery store. They are easy to make and much less expensive.

¼ C	margarine	125 mL
2 t	Amaretto	10 mL
1 t	almond extract	5 mL
2	egg whites	2
8 t	fructose	40 mL
½ C	flour	125 mL
⅓ C	blanched almonds, ground	90 mL

In a small saucepan, melt the margarine; stir in the Amaretto and almond extract. Set aside to cool. In a medium bowl, beat the egg whites until soft peaks form; beat in the fructose, then fold in the flour; beat in the margarine mixture. Mix the almonds into the batter. Drop by small teaspoonfuls onto baking sheets coated with non-stick vegetable cooking spray, spacing mounds well apart. Using a fork dipped in cold water, flatten each mound with a crisscross pattern to make a thin round. Bake in batches in a preheated 450°F (230°C) oven for 5 minutes or until lightly browned around the edges.

Once the cookies are removed from the oven, quickly place them over a rolling pin to give them a gently curved shape.

Yield: 46 cookies   **Exchange:** free
Each cookie contains:
Calories: 23   Fiber: trace
Sodium: 2.3 mg   Cholesterol: 0

Thumb Cookies

Cute and yummy. One of the easiest cookies to make.

1	egg or egg substitute, beaten	1
2 T	skim milk	30 mL
1½ C	flour	375 mL
2 T	sugar	30 mL
3 pkts	concentrated acesulfame-K	3 pkts
2 t	baking powder	10 mL
½ C	margarine or butter	125 mL
1 t	vanilla extract	5 mL
2 T	fruit-only raspberry or strawberry jam	30 mL

In a large bowl, beat together the egg and milk. Remove 1 T and set it aside to be used later. Sift together the dry ingredients. Add the flour mixture, margarine, and vanilla extract to the egg mixture. Mix until thoroughly blended. Roll into balls the size of walnuts. Place the balls on ungreased cookie sheets. Press a thumbprint into the top of each. Fill with jam. Brush the cookies with the egg-and-milk mixture that was set aside previously. Bake at 350°F (180°C) for 10–15 minutes.

Yield: 42 cookies   **Exchange:** ½ bread
     Each cookie contains:
Calories: 45   Fiber: trace
Sodium: 47 mg   Cholesterol: trace

Almond Rusks

This is a traditional Scandinavian recipe. You just make a cake, cut it into fingers, and then toast them until they are crunchy. These are great with coffee or a frozen dessert or even with gelatin.

½ C	margarine or butter	125 mL
¼ C	sugar	60 mL
3 pkts	concentrated acesulfame-K	3 pkts
2 T	nonfat sour cream	30 mL
2	eggs or equivalent egg substitute, lightly beaten	2
1 t	almond extract	5 mL
2 C	flour	500 mL
2 t	baking powder	10 mL
1 C	blanched almonds, chopped fine	250 mL

Cream the margarine, sugar, acesulfame-K, and sour cream. Add the eggs and almond extract. Add the flour, baking powder, and almonds. Spread into an 8½-inch (21 cm) square brownie pan and bake in a 350°F (180°C) oven for 25 minutes or until a cake tester inserted in the center comes out clean. Remove from the oven. Cool the cake in the pan on a wire rack, then turn it out of the pan. Cut the cake in half horizontally. Then cut each half into ¾ × 2-inch (2 × 5 cm) strips. Lay these on an ungreased cookie sheet and brown lightly for about 10 minutes at 350°F (180°C).

Yield: 64 rusks   **Exchange:** ½ fat
     Each rusk contains:
Calories: 43   Fiber: trace
Sodium: 3 mg   Cholesterol: 9 mg

Sweet Potato Cookies

Very moist, soft cookies that are a good way to use up leftover sweet potatoes.

¼ C	sugar	60 mL
3 pkts	concentrated acesulfame-K	3 pkts
¼ C	nonfat cream cheese	60 mL
1 C	sweet potatoes, cooked, mashed	250 mL
¼ C	margarine or butter	60 mL
1	egg or egg substitute	1
2 C	oats	500 mL
1 t	cinnamon	5 mL
½ t	baking soda	2 mL
¼ t	ground cloves	1 mL
1	apple, peeled, cored, and chopped fine	1

Beat together the sugar, acesulfame-K, and cream cheese until smooth. Add all the other ingredients except the chopped apple. Beat the mixture well, then stir the apple in. Drop the batter by tablespoonfuls onto a cookie sheet coated with non-stick cooking spray. With the back of a spoon, press each cookie into a patty. Bake in a 350°F (180°C) oven for about 15–20 minutes. Cool the cookies on a wire rack.

Yield: 50 cookies   **Exchange:** free
Each cookie contains:
Calories: 23   Fiber: trace
Sodium: 18 mg   Cholesterol: 0

Orange Tea Cookies

The Grand Marnier gives these cookies a subtle, rich flavor. You can substitute orange extract if you prefer.

¼ C	margarine or butter	125 mL
1 t	orange extract	5 mL
2 t	Grand Marnier	10 mL
1 t	butter-flavored extract	5 mL
2	egg whites	2
8 t	fructose	40 mL
½ C	all-purpose flour	125 mL
⅓ C	slivered almonds	90 mL

In a small saucepan, melt the margarine; then stir in the orange extract, Grand Marnier, and butter extract. Set aside to cool. In a medium bowl, beat the egg whites until soft peaks form. Add the fructose. Fold in the flour, then beat in the margarine mixture. Mix the almonds into the batter. Drop by small teaspoonfuls onto baking sheets that have been coated with non-stick vegetable cooking spray, spacing mounds well apart. Using a fork dipped in cold water, flatten each mound with a crisscross pattern to make a thin round. Bake in batches in a 450°F (230°C) oven for 5 minutes or until lightly browned around the edges.

Once the cookies are removed from the oven, quickly place them over a rolling pin to give them a gently curved shape.

Yield: 46 cookies   **Exchange:** free
Each cookie contains:
Calories: 22   Fiber: trace
Sodium: 2.3 mg   Cholesterol: 0

Walnut Spice Kisses

This is a meringue cookie and it's easy to make. When the weather is damp, meringue tends to be sticky. They are crisp if the humidity is low.

1	egg white	1
2 dashes	salt	2 dashes
2 T	sugar	30 mL
2 pkts	concentrated acesulfame-K	2 pkts
1 t	cinnamon	5 mL
⅛ t	nutmeg	.5 mL
⅛ t	cloves	.5 mL
1 C	finely chopped walnuts	250 mL
30	walnut halves	30

Beat the egg white until stiff. Gradually beat in the salt. In another bowl, mix the sugar and acesulfame-K with the spices. Beat this into the egg white mixture. Fold in the chopped walnuts. Drop by teaspoonful onto a cookie sheet coated with non-stick cooking spray. Top each cookie with a walnut half. Bake at 250°F (120°C) for 35–40 minutes.

Yield: 30 cookies   **Exchange:** ½ fat
Each cookie contains:
Calories: 32   Fiber: trace
Sodium: 2 mg   Cholesterol: 0

Fruit Tart

A tart has three parts: a delicate tart crust, a creamy filling, and a fruit topping. Although it looks and tastes spectacular, it is not difficult to make. Make up this tart earlier on the day of serving.

Light Tart Crust

½ C	Wondra flour	125 mL
¼ t	baking powder	1.25 mL
¼ C	egg substitute	60 mL
1 t	sugar	5 mL
6 pkts	concentrated acesulfame-K	6 pkts
1 t	vanilla extract	5 mL
1 T	margarine or butter, melted	15 mL

Combine the flour and baking powder. In a separate bowl use an electric mixer to beat the egg substitute, sugar, acesulfame-K, and vanilla extract for a full three minutes. Add the margarine and the flour mixture, then beat. Spoon the mixture evenly onto the bottom of a 9-inch (22.5 cm) springform pan that has been sprayed lightly with non-stick vegetable cooking spray. A good way to spread the dough evenly is to use a rubber spatula to apply it. Push it down firmly and then spread as if you were painting a flat surface.

Place the pan on a cookie sheet and bake it in a preheated 325°F (165°C) oven for 20 minutes. Take the cookie sheet and pan out of the oven. Remove the side from the springform. Then move the crust off its base onto a rack. Place the rack and the crust back on the cookie sheet and bake it an additional 20 minutes. Cool.

Tart Filling

1½ t	flour	7.5 mL
1 T	cornstarch	15 mL
2 pkts	concentrated acesulfame-K	2 pkts
¼ C	egg substitute	60 mL
½ C	skim milk	125 mL
1 t	vanilla extract	5 mL
1 t	concentrated aspartame	5 mL

Use the bowl of an electric mixer to combine the flour, cornstarch, and acesulfame-K. Beat in the egg substitute and heat for two minutes. In a saucepan, bring the milk to the boiling point; then turn off the heat. Slowly pour the hot mixture into the egg-flour mixture and beat briefly to combine. Pour the mixture back into the saucepan, cook for several minutes, whisking constantly. When the mixture has thickened, turn off the heat. Stir in the vanilla extract and the aspartame.

To finish the tart

1 C	raspberries	250 mL
⅔ C	blueberries	180 mL

Spread the tart filling over the tart crust. Then decorate with fruit. Place a ring of raspberries all around the outside edge. Then place the blueberries around the edge but inside the raspberries. There will be approximately six rings of blueberries. Fill in the center with raspberries.

> **Yield:** 8 servings   **Exchange:** 1 bread
> **Each serving contains:**
> Calories: 78   Fiber: 1 g
> Sodium: 57 mg   Cholesterol: trace

Peanut Butter Cookies

As good as Grandma used to make.

2 T	margarine or butter	30 mL
½ C	peanut butter	125 mL
¼ C	sugar	60 mL
3 pkts	concentrated acesulfame-K	3 pkts
1	egg or egg substitute, beaten	1
2 C	flour	500 mL
4 t	baking powder	20 mL
⅓ C	milk	90 mL

Cream the margarine thoroughly, add the peanut butter and cream together, then blend in the sugar and acesulfame-K. Add the beaten egg. Mix and sift the dry ingredients and add them alternately to the creamed mixture with the milk. Roll into small balls and place on a baking sheet coated with non-stick cooking spray. Flatten with the bottom of a glass dipped in flour. Then, using a fork, make criss-cross impressions in each cookie. Bake in a 400°F (200°C) oven for 7 minutes.

> **Yield:** 70 cookies   **Exchange:** free
> **Each cookie contains:**
> Calories: 27   Fiber: trace
> Sodium: 37 mg   Cholesterol: 0

Coconut Kisses

If you love coconut, you'll love these easy-to-make cookies.

¼ t	salt	1 mL
½ C	egg whites	125 mL
¼ C	sugar	60 mL
6 pkts	concentrated acesulfame-K	6 pkts
½ t	vanilla extract	2 mL
2½ C	shredded coconut	625 mL

Add the salt to the egg whites and beat until foamy. Gradually beat in the sugar and acesulfame-K. Beat until the egg whites are stiff. Fold in the vanilla extract and coconut.

Drop by teaspoonfuls onto cookie sheets coated with non-stick cooking spray. Leave about 2 inches (3 cm) between cookies for spreading. Bake in a 325°F (160°C) oven for 20 minutes. The cookies will be light brown. Cool on wire racks.

Yield: 50 cookies **Exchange:** free
Each cookie contains:
Calories: 22 Fiber: trace
Sodium: 10 mg Cholesterol: 0

Crisp Oat Cookies

Crisp cookies that store well.

⅓ C	margarine or butter	90 mL
⅓ C	nonfat cream cheese	90 mL
¼ C	sugar	90 mL
3 pkts	concentrated acesulfame-K	3 pkts
3 C	oatmeal	750 mL

Beat together the margarine, cream cheese, sugar, and acesulfame-K. Mix in the oatmeal until well blended. Roll the dough into small balls. Place each ball on a cookie sheet sprayed with non-stick cooking spray. Flatten the balls crosswise with a fork. Bake in a 350°F (180°C) oven until light brown, about 8 minutes.

Yield: 50 cookies **Exchange:** ½ bread
Each cookie contains:
Calories: 67 Fiber: trace
Sodium: 7 mg Cholesterol: trace

Pecan Tea Cookies

These cookies are rolled into balls, so they are fast to make. Everyone will love them.

2 C	finely chopped pecans	500 mL
1 C	margarine	250 mL
2 T	sugar	30 mL
2 pkts	concentrated acesulfame-K	2 pkts
2 C	flour	500 mL
1 t	vanilla extract	5 mL
1 T	water	15 mL

Mix all the ingredients together. Chill for half an hour. Shape into small balls. Place on a cookie sheet coated with non-stick cooking spray. Bake in a 350°F (180°C) oven for 12–13 minutes until light brown.

Yield: 80 cookies   **Exchange:** 1 fat
Each cookie contains:
Calories: 50   Fiber: trace
Sodium: trace   Cholesterol: 0

Rice Krispies-and-Date Squares

These are yummy beyond belief. Hint: Use a sharp, wet knife to cut the dates.

¾ C	chopped dates	190 mL
2 T	margarine	30 mL
1	egg or egg substitute, slightly beaten	1
1 T	nonfat milk	15 mL
1 t	vanilla extract	5 mL
4 pkts	concentrated aspartame	4 pkts
3 C	toasted rice cereal	750 mL

Mix the chopped dates, margarine, egg, milk, and vanilla extract in a medium saucepan. Cook over medium heat until thick, about five minutes. Cool, then stir in the aspartame and cereal. Press into an 8-inch (20 cm) square pan coated with non-stick cooking spray. Refrigerate until firm. Cut into 24 squares.

Yield: 24 squares   **Exchange:** ½ bread
Each square contains:
Calories: 36   Fiber: trace
Sodium: 55 mg   Cholesterol: 0

Fudgy Brownies

Prune puree eliminates all fat and it makes these brownies seem like sinful fudge.

1½ C	apple juice, unsweetened	375 mL
½ C	Prune Puree (page 138)	125 mL
4	egg whites	4
1 t	vanilla extract	5 mL
1 t	chocolate extract	5 mL
1 C	flour	250 mL
¼ C	measures-like-sugar saccharin	60 mL
⅔ C	unsweetened cocoa powder	180 mL
2 t	baking powder	30 mL
½ t	baking soda	2 mL

Mix the apple juice, prune puree, egg whites, and vanilla and chocolate extracts. Sift together the remaining ingredients and gradually add the flour mixture to the wet mixture. Use an electric mixer to blend. Pour into a 9-inch (23 cm) square baking pan coated with non-stick cooking spray. Bake in a preheated 350°F (180°C) oven for 30 minutes. Cool and cut into squares.

Yield: 16 brownies   **Exchange:** ½ bread
Each brownie contains:
Calories: 49   Fiber: trace
Sodium: 122 mg   Cholesterol: 0

Cakelike Brownies

These are a favorite for people who like a lighter-textured brownie.

1 C	sifted flour	250 mL
½ C	unsweetened cocoa powder	125 mL
pinch	salt (optional)	pinch
¼ t	baking powder	1 mL
¼ t	baking soda	1 mL
3 T	margarine or butter	45 mL
2 T	Prune Puree (page 138)	30 mL
2 T	sugar	30 mL
20 pkts	concentrated acesulfame-K	20 pkts
¼ C	nonfat, sugar-free, plain yogurt	60 mL
½ C	egg substitute or 2 eggs	125 mL
1 t	vanilla extract	5 mL

Sift the first five ingredients together twice; set aside. Melt the margarine or butter in a saucepan over low heat. Add the prune puree and combine with a wire whisk. Turn off the heat; add sugar and acesulfame-K and mix well. Add the yogurt, egg substitute, and vanilla extract and stir with a wire whisk. Add the flour mixture and stir with a large spoon to combine. Pour the mixture into an 8-inch (20 cm) square baking pan that has been coated with non-stick cooking spray. Bake in a preheated 350°F (180°C) oven for 25 minutes. When cool, cut into 16 squares.

Yield: 16 squares   **Exchange:** ½ bread
  Each square contains:
Calories: 69   Fiber: trace
Sodium: 60 mg   Cholesterol: 0

Brownies

This version will make the most discriminating brownie eater happy.

½ C	sugar	125 mL
2 t	concentrated saccharin	10 g
⅓ C	flour	90 mL
⅓ C	unsweetened cocoa powder	90 mL
1 t	baking soda	5 mL
¼ C	canola oil	60 mL
2	eggs	2
2 t	butter-flavored extract	10 mL
1 t	vanilla extract	5 mL

In one bowl combine the dry ingredients. In another bowl combine the wet ingredients. Stir the wet ingredients into the dry ones. Pour the batter into an 8-inch (20 cm) square brownie pan coated with non-stick cooking spray, and bake in a 350°F (180°C) oven for 25 minutes. Cool on a wire rack.

Yield: 16 brownies   **Exchange:** ½ bread + ½ fat
  Each brownie contains:
Calories: 81   Fiber: trace
Sodium: 108 mg   Cholesterol: 19 mg

Apple Squares

These squares travel well and are moist and delicious. In addition, they are quick and easy to make. The hard part is waiting for them to cool!

6 pkts	concentrated acesulfame-K	6 pkts
1 C	flour, sifted	250 mL
1 t	baking soda	5 mL
1 t	cinnamon	5 mL
1	egg or equivalent egg substitute	1
¼ C	canola oil	60 mL
2 t	vanilla extract	10 mL
2 C	apples, peeled, cored, chopped	500 mL
2 T	water	30 mL

Sift together the acesulfame-K, flour, baking soda, and cinnamon. Mix the egg, oil, and vanilla extract in a separate bowl. Add to the flour mixture. Using an electric mixer, beat at medium speed until well blended (the mixture will be stiff). Add the apple mixture and water. Mix well. Pour into an 8-inch- (20 cm) square pan coated with non-stick cooking spray.

Bake in a 350°F (180°C) oven for 25 minutes or until a toothpick tests clean. Cool 10 minutes; then cut into squares.

Yield: 16 squares   **Exchange:** 1 bread + ½ fat
Each square contains:
Calories: 76   Fiber: trace
Sodium: 79 mg   Cholesterol: 0

Banana Squares

Try these squares when you're looking to make something a little out of the ordinary.

⅓ C	nonfat dry milk	90 mL
⅓ C	ice water	90 mL
3	eggs or egg substitute	3
4 pkts	concentrated acesulfame-K	4 pkts
3 T	margarine	45 mL
2 t	instant coffee powder	10 mL
1 t	vanilla extract	5 mL
1½ C	flour	375 mL
1½ t	baking powder	7 mL
½ t	baking soda	2 mL
2 C	mashed bananas (2)	500 mL

Whip the dry milk and ice water until stiff peaks form. In another bowl, beat the eggs until thick and lemon-colored. To the eggs, add the acesulfame-K, margarine, coffee, and vanilla. Sift together the flour, baking powder, and baking soda. Stir the flour mixture into the egg mixture. Add the bananas. Fold the whipped dry milk into the batter. Spread the batter evenly in a 9-inch (23 cm) pan coated with non-stick cooking spray. Bake in a 375°F (190°C) oven for 25–30 minutes or until the cake tests done.

Yield: 16 squares		**Exchange:** 1 bread
Each square contains:		
Calories: 89		Fiber: trace
Sodium: 99 mg		Cholesterol: trace

Spice Squares

These squares taste like old-fashioned spice cake delivered in snack form.

¼ C	measures-like-sugar saccharin	60 mL
¼ C	sugar	60 mL
3 pkts	concentrated acesulfame-K	3 pkts
2	eggs or egg substitute	2
2 C	flour	500 mL
½ t	baking soda	7 mL
½ t	cloves	7 mL
½ t	allspice	7 mL
1 t	cinnamon	5 mL
½ C	chopped raisins	125 mL
½ C	chopped dates	125 mL
½ C	nuts (optional)	125 mL
½ C	strong coffee	125 mL

Add the saccharin, sugar, and acesulfame-K to the eggs and beat until light and foamy. Sift the dry ingredients together, add the chopped raisins, dates, and nuts, and combine with the creamed mixture alternately with the coffee. Spread the mixture ½ inch (1.5 cm) thick in a 9 × 13-inch (23 × 33 cm) lasagna pan coated with non-stick cooking spray and bake in a preheated 400°F (200°C) oven for 30 minutes. When cool, cut into squares.

Yield: 24 squares		**Exchange:** 1 bread
Each square contains:		
Calories: 69		Fiber: trace
Sodium: 35 mg		Cholesterol: 0

Sour Cream–Fruit Refrigerator Squares

This is a fancy gelatin variation. Make it up on a hot afternoon and enjoy it in the cool of the evening.

1 pkg	sugar-free strawberry gelatin	1 pkg
1½ C	boiling water	375 mL
1 C	cold water	250 mL
	ice cubes	
1 T	lemon juice	15 mL
½ C	nonfat sour cream	125 mL
1 (8 oz.) can	pears, no sugar added, drained and coarsely chopped	1 (250 mL) can

In a large bowl, dissolve the gelatin in boiling water. Combine the cold water and ice cubes to make 2½ C (625 mL). Add to the gelatin and stir until slightly thickened, then remove any unmelted ice.

Measure and remove 1½ C (375 mL) of the gelatin mixture, add lemon juice, and set aside. Blend the sour cream into the remaining gelatin and pour it into a 8-inch (20 cm) square pan coated with non-stick cooking spray. Carefully arrange the fruit on the creamy gelatin, then spoon clear gelatin over the top. Chill until firm, about three hours. Cut into squares.

Yield: 9 squares **Exchange:** ½ fruit
Each square contains:
Calories: 30   Fiber: trace
Sodium: 42 mg   Cholesterol: 1.8 mg

Lemon Squares

These are everybody's favorite—as close as can be to the high-sugar ones you are most probably familiar with.

Crust

1 C	flour	250 mL
¼ t	baking soda	1 mL
¼ t	baking powder	1 mL
pinch	salt (optional)	pinch
2 T	margarine or butter	30 mL
½ t	butter-flavored extract	2 mL
2 t	sugar	10 mL
4 pkts	concentrated acesulfame-K	4 pkts
1 t	vanilla extract	5 mL
1 t	fresh lemon peel	5 mL
⅓ C	egg substitute	90 mL

¼ C	nonfat sour cream	60 mL

Filling

⅓ C	egg substitute	90 mL
1 T	sugar	15 mL
6 pkts	concentrated acesulfame-K	6 pkts
¼ C	cornstarch	60 mL
2 t	lemon peel	10 mL
½ C	lemon juice	125 mL

Glaze

1 T	concentrated aspartame	15 mL
2 T	boiling water	30 mL
2 t	cornstarch	10 mL

To make the crust, sift together the first four ingredients and set aside. Using an electric mixer, soften the margarine, then add the butter extract, sugar, acesulfame-K, vanilla extract, and lemon peel. Beat to combine. Beat in the egg substitute and sour cream. Add the flour mixture and combine. Spread the dough into the bottom of an 8-inch (20 cm) square baking pan that has been sprayed with non-stick vegetable cooking spray. Have patience; the batter will be thick and it will take a little effort to spread it out easily. Bake in a preheated 325°F (160°C) oven for 20 minutes.

While the crust is baking, make the filling. Combine the egg substitute, sugar, and acesulfame-K and beat with an electric mixer. Add the cornstarch, lemon peel, and lemon juice, and beat briefly to combine. Remove the crust from the oven when it is lightly browned. Pour in the egg-lemon mixture. Return the crust to the oven for 20 minutes.

After it is out of the oven, mix the glaze. Combine the boiling water, cornstarch, and aspartame. Poke holes in many places in the top. With a pastry brush spread the glaze evenly over the top. Chill. Cut into 16 squares.

Yield: 16 squares   **Exchange:** 1 bread
Each square contains:
Calories: 63   Fiber: trace
Sodium: 50 mg   Cholesterol: trace

Chocolate Muffins

Great to make for people who need to be reminded to eat only a single portion. Make them, freeze them, and defrost as needed.

½ C	unsweetened cocoa powder	125 mL
1 C	flour	250 mL
1 t	baking soda	5 mL
½ t	baking powder	2 mL
pinch	salt (optional)	pinch
2 T	sugar	30 mL
½ C	fructose	125 mL
4 pkts	concentrated acesulfame-K	4 pkts
1 C	nonfat buttermilk	250 mL
½ C	prune puree	125 mL
2 t	vanilla extract	10 mL
¼ t	almond extract	1 mL
2	egg whites	2

Glaze

2 t	unsweetened cocoa powder	10 mL
	hot water	
¼ C	measures-like-sugar aspartame	60 mL

Sift the cocoa, flour, baking soda, baking powder, salt, sugar, fructose, and acesulfame-K together twice. Set aside. Use a food processor to combine the buttermilk, prune puree, vanilla, and almond extract. Add the dry ingredients and process briefly. Transfer to a mixing bowl. Beat the egg whites until stiff. Stir the egg whites into the batter.

Pour the batter into 18 muffin tin cups that have been coated with nonstick cooking spray. Bake in a preheated 325°F (160°C) oven for 20 minutes. Combine the glaze with a wire whisk. Pour a little glaze over each muffin.

Yield: 18 muffins   **Exchange:** 1 bread
Each muffin contains:
Calories: 70   Fiber: trace
Sodium: 108 mg   Cholesterol: 0

Blueberry Muffins

Almost every doughnut shop and breakfast restaurant now sells blueberry muffins. A generous size of muffin has become the standard in restaurants and bakeries. However, the size specified in cookbooks, especially diabetic cookbooks, is a miniature version. We hope you won't be disappointed that we are calling for the old-fashioned small size. You can use a standard cupcake pan or paper liners.

1½ C	flour	375 mL
1½ t	baking powder	7 mL
¼ t	baking soda	1 mL
1 T	canola oil	15 mL
⅓ C	egg substitute	90 mL
½ C	nonfat buttermilk	125 mL
½ t	vanilla extract	2 mL
2 T	nonfat sour cream	30 mL
¼ C	apple juice concentrate	60 mL
1 C	blueberries (fresh or frozen without sugar and defrosted)	250 mL
3 T	boiling water	45 mL
2 t	concentrated aspartame	10 mL

Sift together the flour, baking powder, and baking soda. Set aside. Use a wire whisk to combine the oil, egg substitute, buttermilk, vanilla extract, sour cream, and apple juice concentrate. Stir the flour mixture into the wet mixture. Do not overmix. Stir in the blueberries. Pour into a muffin tin that has been coated with non-stick cooking spray.

Bake in a preheated 375°F (190°C) oven for 30 minutes. As soon as the muffins are out of the oven, combine the boiling water and aspartame to make a glaze. Use a toothpick to make holes in the tops of the muffins. Use a pastry brush to cover the tops with the glaze.

Yield: 12 muffins   **Exchange:** 1 bread
Each muffin contains:
Calories: 90   Fiber: trace
Sodium: 100 mg   Cholesterol: trace

Low-Calorie Lemon–Poppy Seed Muffins

These muffins are high in flavor and low in calories. They are great as a dessert or as a snack with coffee or tea.

1 C	nonfat cottage cheese	250 mL
¼ C	egg substitute	60 mL
¼ C	flour	60 mL
1 t	vanilla extract	5 mL
2 t	lemon juice	10 mL
2 t	grated lemon peel	10 mL
1 T	sugar	15 mL
2 pkts	concentrated acesulfame-K	2 pkts
2 t	poppy seed	10 mL
4 drops	yellow food coloring	4 drops
2	egg whites	2
⅛ t	cream of tartar	.35 mL
3 T	boiling water	45 mL
1 T	measures-like-sugar aspartame	15 mL

Put the cottage cheese into a food processor or blender; process for a few minutes until very smooth. Add the egg substitute, flour, vanilla extract, lemon juice, lemon peel. sugar, acesulfame-K, poppy seed, and food coloring. Process until well combined. Use an electric mixer to beat the egg whites until they hold their peaks; add the cream of tartar and continue beating until soft. Add a small amount of the blended egg whites into the food processor and combine. Then pour the mixture from the food processor into another mixing bowl. Gently fold the rest of the beaten egg whites into the batter using a rubber spatula.

Pour approximately ¼ C (60 mL) of batter into a muffin pan that has been sprayed with non-stick vegetable cooking spray. Bake in preheated 300°F (155°C) oven for 20 minutes. As soon as the muffins are out of the oven, combine the boiling water and aspartame to make the glaze. Use a fork to poke holes in the tops of the muffins. Pour the glaze into the holes.

Yield: 14 muffins   **Exchange:** free
Each muffin contains:
Calories: 29   Fiber: trace
Sodium: 17 mg   Cholesterol: 1 mg

CHAPTER FIVE

Pies and Turnovers

Missing from most discussions of pie is an honest acknowledgment of how high the fat content is. One small slice of a traditional two-crust pie has more than three fat exchanges, and that's just the crust. These numbers assume that a standard nine-inch pie is cut into eight slices. If you eat one-sixth of a two-crust pie, you get *four* fat exchanges, again for just the crust portion.

What to do about this depressing pie crust news? We give you many choices in pie crusts, ranging from a totally fat-free meringue to a traditional pie crust. It's up to you to decide how many calories and fat exchanges you are willing to spend on pie crust. We're following current standard practice in stating that one serving is one-eighth of a nine-inch pie.

We list the recipes for crusts separate from the recipes for fillings. You decide which crust you wish to pair with which filling. Be sure to combine the calories, exchanges, etc., for the total.

For our meringue pie crust, the crust portion of one slice is only 30 calories. There is no fat or cholesterol, and there are no exchanges. The trade-off is that with a meringue pie crust, you have to plan ahead and give it time to cook and cool, although it is very easy to do. Another trade-off is that a meringue pie crust can be unexciting.

Next best, in terms of fat and calorie scores, is the cottage cheese–based pie crust. One slice of this crust has only 52 calories and 2.8 grams of fat, for half a fat exchange.

Next best is our graham cracker crust. One slice is only 86 calories and 2.2 grams of fat, also half a fat exchange. We made our graham cracker crust with nonfat cream cheese instead of margarine or butter.

Next comes a flour-based pie crust in which we used half margarine and half nonfat cream cheese. One slice of a pie with a bottom crust only has 97 calories and 4.3 grams of fat. It looks beautiful, but we must be honest and tell you that it is not as flaky as Grandmom's pie crust made with (unhealthy) lard.

When we use all margarine for our flour-based pie crust, one slice of bottom-crust-only pie has 140 calories and 8.5 grams of fat. A slice from a pie with a top and bottom crust has 241 calories and 15.5 grams of fat. All these figures are for the crust portion only.

We do have some other crust suggestions. You can use fillo dough to make a nice top crust; the cost per slice is low in calories. We do not recommend using fillo dough for a bottom crust; the dough dissolves into an unattractive goo. The idea of putting a fruit filling into an empty pie pan and then covering it with fillo dough may seem strange when you first hear about it. But it works quite well. Our taste testers liked the pies with just a fillo-dough top crust. And it costs almost nothing in calories.

A turnover is like a little pie. We offer a couple of suggestions to get you started. You can substitute any other appropriate filling.

Fat-Free Pie Crust

This is basically an egg-white meringue, so it has very few calories. It's easy to make and looks quite impressive. It's best to make the crust the day before you fill it and serve it. Keep in mind that meringues get sticky in damp weather.

1 C	egg whites	250 mL
1 t	vanilla extract	5 mL
6 pkts	concentrated acesulfame-K	6 pkts
¼ t	cream of tartar	1 mL
1 T	sugar	15 mL

Using an electric mixer, beat the egg whites until foamy, then add the vanilla extract, acesulfame-K, cream of tartar and sugar. Pour the mixture into a 9-inch (23 cm) pie pan that has been coated with non-stick cooking spray. Use a spatula to distribute the mixture evenly into a pie crust shape. Bake in a preheated 250°F (120°C) oven for one hour. Turn off the heat and let the pie crust cool in the oven.

Yield: 8 servings   **Exchange:** free
Each serving contains:
Calories: 30   Fiber: 0
Sodium: 86 mg   Cholesterol: 0

Cottage Cheese Pie Crust

You'll be pleased with this pie crust. It's low-calorie and virtually foolproof.

⅓ C	flour, sifted	60 mL
2 T	margarine	30 mL
½ C	nonfat cottage cheese	125 mL

Drain the cottage cheese dry, then place it in a food processor with a metal blade and blend until pureed. Discard any liquid. Cut the margarine into the dry ingredients as you would for a regular pie crust, then add the cottage cheese, mixing lightly with a fork until a ball of dough is formed. Turn onto a lightly floured pastry cloth and roll it to fit an 8-inch (20 cm) or 9-inch (23 cm) pie pan coated with nonfat cooking spray. Prick the crust all over with a fork.

Yield: 8 servings   **Exchange:** ½ fat
Each serving contains:
Calories: 52   Fiber: trace
Sodium: 32.3 mg   Cholesterol: 1.3 mg

Buttery Graham Cracker Crust

Using nonfat cream cheese instead of margarine or butter reduces the fat dramatically as compared to the traditional version.

1¼ C	graham cracker crumbs	310 mL
2 oz.	nonfat cream cheese	56 g
1 t	butter-flavored extract	5 mL
½ t	cinnamon	2 mL

Combine the ingredients in a food processor. Use your fingers or a spoon to press the mixture firmly into a 9-inch (23 cm) pie pan. Bake at 325°F (160°C) for 8 to 10 minutes.

Yield: 8 servings   **Exchange:** 1 bread
Each serving contains:
Calories: 86   Fiber: trace
Sodium: 133 mg   Cholesterol: 3 mg

One-Crust Pastry Pie Crust for a Nine-Inch (23 cm) Shell

Here we used part margarine and part nonfat cream cheese for a pretty good pie crust. Although it's not as flaky as Grandmom's crust made with (unbelievably) lard, its fat and calorie content are acceptable.

1 C	flour	250 mL
3 T	margarine	45 mL
3 T	nonfat cream cheese	45 mL
3 T	ice water	45 mL
1 T	flour	15 mL

Combine all the ingredients using a pastry blender or process in a food processor for a few seconds. With your hands, firm the dough into a ball. Chill the dough in the refrigerator for at least half an hour.

Sprinkle a small amount of flour on a countertop or large wooden board. Center the dough on the floured surface. Roll the dough into a circle slightly larger than the pie pan. Carefully lift the pie crust into the pan. If it will be baked unfilled, use a fork to prick the bottom and sides. Bake in a preheated 375°F (190°C) oven for 8–9 minutes.

Yield: 8 servings   **Exchange:** 1 bread + ½ fat
Each serving contains:
Calories: 97   Fiber: trace
Sodium: 74 mg   Cholesterol: trace

Traditional Pie Crusts

We decided to include a classic pastry pie crust so you can compare the numbers with the low-fat ones we developed for you. We've included a two-crust pie crust and a one-crust pie crust. Follow the same directions for both.

Crust for two-crust pie

2 C	flour	500 mL
11 T	unsalted margarine	170 mL
⅓ C	ice water	90 mL

Crust for one-crust pie

1¼ C	flour	310 mL
6 T	unsalted margarine	90 mL
3 T	ice water	5 mL

Put the flour into a bowl. Using two knives or a pastry blender, cut in the margarine until the mixture resembles coarse meal. Add about two tablespoons (30 mL) of water and work it gently with a fork. Gradually add and mix in the rest of the water, using your fingers or a pastry blender to work the dough into a ball. Chill the dough for 30 minutes. If you are in a hurry, proceed to the next step immediately. If there is enough dough for two crusts, divide the dough roughly in half and keep half in the refrigerator while you roll the first crust.

On a lightly floured surface, flatten the dough into a circle with roundish edges. Use a rolling pin to roll the dough into a circle slightly bigger than the pie pan, rolling from the center outward. Fold the circle of dough in half and gently lift it onto the pie pan, being careful not to stretch it. Unfold the dough and pat it gently into the pan. Using a kitchen knife, cut off any extra dough that is more than ¾ inch (3 cm) beyond the edge of the pan. Fold the outside dough over to make a double thickness of dough around the rim of the pan. Press the dough edge down with a fork, or use your fingers to make a fluted edge. If the crust will be baked without any filling, prick the crust all over with a fork.

Bake in a 425°F (220°C) oven for approximately 12–15 minutes or until it is lightly browned.

> **Yield:** 8 servings of crust for two-crust pie
> **Exchange:** 3 fat + 1½ bread
> **Each serving contains:**
> Calories: 241   Fiber: trace
> Sodium: 178 mg   Cholesterol: 0

Graham Cracker Crust for a Ten-Inch (25 cm) Pie

This is like the recipe often found on the graham cracker box.

1½ C	graham cracker crumbs (18 squares)	375 mL
3 pkts	concentrated acesulfame-K	3 pkts
⅓ C	margarine or butter, melted	90 mL

Mix the graham cracker crumbs and acesulfame-K together in a bowl. Add the margarine and mix thoroughly. Press firmly and evenly into the bottom and sides of a pie pan. Bake in a 350°F (180°C) oven for 10 minutes. Cool before adding the filling.

> **Yield:** 10 servings   **Exchange:** ½ bread + 1 fat
> **Each serving contains:**
> Calories: 106   Fiber: trace
> Sodium: 81 mg   Cholesterol: 0

Graham Cracker Crust for an Eight-Inch (20 cm) Pie

Use this recipe for a small pie pan.

1¼ C	graham cracker crumbs (15 squares)	310 mL
2 pkts	concentrated acesulfame-K	2 pkts
¼ C	margarine or butter	60 mL

Follow the directions for a 10-inch (25 cm) pie, above.

Yield: 8 servings   **Exchange:** ½ bread + 1 fat
Each serving contains:
Calories: 106   Fiber: trace
Sodium: 86 mg   Cholesterol: 0

Fillo Dough

Greek fillo dough is low in fat and calories and it's easy to use to make pie shells, individual tarts, napoleons, or turnovers. Most grocery stores sell frozen packages. Defrosted dough may be kept in the refrigerator for a few weeks.

To use fillo, bring the dough to room temperature. Arrange two surfaces to work on, one for the current sheet and one to store the balance. Take out sheets of fillo only as needed.

While working on one, be careful to keep the others moist. Fillo dough dries out quickly when uncovered, so have all the equipment and ingredients ready before taking the dough out of the package. Using plastic wrap, cover the sheets you are not currently using. A large, clean, plastic-wastebasket-size bag works better than two narrow sheets of plastic wrap. Place a damp dish towel over the plastic, taking care that the towel does not touch the dough and cause it to fall apart. Discard any problem sheets.

Instructions accompanying fillo suggest covering each layer with softened butter. But using a butter-flavored non-stick cooking spray works well.

Yield: a sheet of dough is one serving   **Exchange:** 2 breads
Each sheet contains:
Calories: 180   Fiber: 1 g
Sodium: 120 mg   Cholesterol: 0

Fillo Top Crust for a Nine-Inch (23-cm) Pie

Fillo dough can be used to make an attractive top crust with few calories and little fat. Put your choice of pie filling into a pie pan with no bottom crust.

4 sheets	fillo dough	4 sheets
	butter-flavored non-stick cooking spray	

Place one large sheet of dough on a dry surface. Spray lightly with non-stick cooking spray. Put a second sheet on top. Place a 9-inch (23 cm) metal pie pan face-up in the center of the top layer of the double layer of dough. Spray again. Use scissors to cut away any dough that sticks out more than one inch (2.5 cm) around the edge of the pan. Carefully lift this dough up over the top of the filled pie shell. Use scissors to cut off excess dough, more than one inch (2.5 cm) around edge. Use your fingers to form the edge into a fluted pie shell. Spray lightly with non-stick cooking spray. Bake in a pre-heated 375°F (190°C) oven for seven minutes or until nicely browned.

Tart Shells

Fillo pastry tarts may be available in your supermarket; if not, use this recipe.

Put four sheets of fillo dough on a work surface. Cut a few inches from one side to form squares. Cut each of these squares into four pieces, making 16 small squares.

Take one square and lay it flat. Coat it with non-stick cooking spray. Place another square on top of it, catercorner, forming an eight-pointed star. Carefully press it to the inside or outside a tart pan or custard cup that has been sprayed with non-stick cooking spray. Press the dough against the inside of a 6-ounce (188 g) custard cup to make a tart shell that can hold ½ C (120 mL) of filling. Leave the cup in place to protect the delicate shell.

Repeat to make seven other shells. Place them on a cookie sheet, not touching. Bake in a preheated 375°F (190°C) oven for 8–9 minutes. When the dough is golden brown, remove turnovers from the oven and let cool for a few minutes. Carefully lift the fillo shells from the custard cups or the tart pan and allow to finish cooling on a wire rack. Before serving, fill with your choice of filling. Good choices include fresh or frozen berries, defrosted (sprinkled with a little aspartame or acesulfame-K, if desired); pudding (vanilla or chocolate, no-sugar, no-fat, instant mixes or other recipes, such as the ones in the pudding chapter); a thin layer of vanilla pudding plus fruit; sugar-free, fat-free frozen yogurt

These tarts are not good finger food: as they are so thin, they shatter easily. But eaten with a fork or spoon, they are elegant and seem self-indulgent despite their low calories and low fat.

Creamy Prune Pie Filling

The combination of prunes, lemon flavor, and cardamom makes a special "European" dish.

10 pkts	concentrated acesulfame-K	10 packets
⅓ C	flour	90 mL
pinch	salt (optional)	pinch
2 C	skim milk	500 mL
⅓ C	egg substitute	90 mL
1 C	nonfat sour cream	250 mL
1 t	vanilla extract	5 mL
2 t	grated lemon peel	10 mL
1 t	lemon juice	5 mL
½ C	pitted prunes, cut into small pieces	125 mL

Topping

3	egg whites	3
¼ t	cream of tartar	1.25 mL
2 t	sugar	10 mL
3 pkts	concentrated acesulfame-K	3 pkts
½ t	cardamom	2.5 mL

Combine the 10 packets of acesulfame-K, flour, and salt in a saucepan. Add the milk and stir to combine. Bring to a boil and cook for 1–2 minutes, stirring with a wire whisk. Turn off the heat. In a separate container, add a small amount of the hot milk and the egg substitute. Return this to the saucepan and cook for several minutes over low heat, stirring with a wire whisk. Let cool for a few minutes. Add the sour cream, vanilla extract, lemon peel, lemon juice, and prune pieces. Whisk together. Pour into a prepared pie shell or into an empty 9-inch (23 cm) pan if you wish to reduce calories.

Then prepare the topping. Beat the egg whites with an electric mixer, add in the cream of tartar near the end. Then beat in the sugar, acesulfame-K, and cardamom. Spread the meringue over the top of the pie. Use a rubber spatula to be sure the topping goes all the way to the edges. Bake in a preheated 350°F (180°C) oven for 13 minutes. Cool in the refrigerator.

Yield: 8 servings **Exchange:** 1 milk
Each serving contains:
Calories: 97 Fiber: trace
Sodium: 110 mg Cholesterol: 5 mg

Not-Quite-American Apple (or Cherry) Pie

This is an example of how to combine a dough or crust recipe with a filling recipe.

4 pieces	fillo dough	4 pieces
4 C	apple or cherry filling (from this book)	1 L

First make the fruit filling, following the directions on page 77 or 78. Turn the filling into a 9-inch (23 cm) pie pan that has been coated with non-stick vegetable cooking spray. Set aside. Following the general instructions for using fillo dough, spread one sheet of dough onto a work surface and coat it with cooking spray. Spread the second sheet of dough over the first. Spray. Repeat until there are four layers on top of one another. Lift these four layers together and center them over the fruit-filled pie pan. Use a pair of clean scissors to trim away all but one inch (2.5 cm) around the edge of the dough. Use your fingers to crimp together the edge to reassemble a traditional pie crust. Bake in a preheated 375°F (190°C) oven for 15 minutes or until the top is nicely browned. Watch carefully that it does not overcook.

Yield: 8 servings

Apple Pie Filling for Pie or Tarts

The sweetness of the filling depends on the type of apple you choose.

4 C	apple, peeled, sliced thin	1 L
1 T	cinnamon	15 mL
1 t	nutmeg	5 mL
1 T	vanilla extract	15 mL
2 T	lemon juice	30 mL
6 pkts	concentrated acesulfame-K	6 pkts
1 t	grated lemon peel	5 mL

Put the apple slices into a large non-stick pan that has been coated with non-stick cooking spray. Cover and cook for about 10 minutes. Stir occasionally. When the apple slices are soft, add the remaining ingredients and stir to mix.

This recipe makes enough for one 9-inch (23 cm) pie or 12 tarts.

Yield: 8 servings   **Exchange:** 1½ fruit
Each serving contains:
Calories: 89   Fiber: 4 g
Sodium: 1 mg   Cholesterol: 0

Apple Prune Pie Filling

You can make a traditional pie by spooning this filling into an unbaked pastry shell and topping it with another crust. To cut way down on fat and calories, spoon the filling into an empty pie pan and top it with a fillo dough crust.

1 C	prunes	250 mL
¾ C	apple juice, unsweetened	190 mL
2 t	finely grated lemon peel	10 mL
2 T	applejack liqueur (optional)	30 mL
6	apples, peeled and sliced	6
1 t	vanilla extract	5 mL
1 t	lemon juice	5 mL
1 t	cinnamon	5 mL
½ t	nutmeg	2 mL
2 T	flour	30 mL
2 T	measures-like-sugar saccharin	30 mL

Combine the first four ingredients in a small saucepan; simmer for a few minutes, then turn off the heat. In a separate bowl, combine the apples and the remaining ingredients. Puree the prune mixture in a blender or food processor. Combine with the apple mixture. Spoon into a prepared crust, if desired. Top with a second crust. Bake in a 425°F (220°C) oven for 10 minutes. Turn the heat down to 350°F (180°C) and bake for an additional 40 minutes. Cool on a wire rack.

Yield: 8 servings   **Exchange:** 2 fruits
Each serving contains:
Calories: 106   Fiber: 4 g
Sodium: 2 mg   Cholesterol: 0

Cherry Pie Filling

Be sure to buy cherries packed in water or juice with no sugar.

2 (14.5 oz.) cans	cherries, in water	2 (411 g) cans
3 T	quick-cooking tapioca	45 mL
5 pkts	concentrated acesulfame-K	5 pkts
¼ t	almond extract	1 mL
5 drops	red food coloring	5 drops
1 t	lemon peel	5 mL

Drain the cherries, reserving ⅓ C (90 mL) of the liquid. Whisk together all the remaining ingredients, then let the mixture thicken for 15 minutes. Use a two-crust pastry recipe for the crust or use the fillo recipe below.

To make a cherry pie with a fillo dough crust, follow the general instructions for fillo dough. Spread out one layer and coat it with non-stick cooking spray. Top it with a second layer, and spray. Repeat until there are four layers on top of one another. Lift the dough onto the fruit in the pie pan. Coat with non-stick cooking spray. Use scissors to trim away all but one inch (2.5 cm) around the edge. Use your fingers to crimp it in to form an edge. Bake in a preheated 375°F (190°C) oven for 15 minutes.

Yield: 8 servings   **Exchange:** 1 fruit
Each serving contains:
Calories: 55   Fiber: trace
Sodium: 1.3 mg   Cholesterol: 0

Lemon Chiffon Pie Filling

If you like a light, tart lemon chiffon pie, this easy recipe is for you. It's perfect on a hot summer evening. Our friend Marge thinks it's wonderful after a lobster dinner.

1 env.	unflavored gelatin	1 env.
6 pkts	concentrated acesulfame-K	6 pkts
4	eggs, separated	4
½ C	lemon juice (fresh is best)	125 mL
¼ C	water	60 mL

Thoroughly mix the gelatin and three packs of acesulfame-K in the top of a double boiler. Beat together the egg yolks, lemon juice, and water; add this to the gelatin.

Cook the mixture over boiling water, stirring constantly until the gelatin is dissolved, about 5 minutes. Remove from the heat. Chill, stirring occasionally until the mixture mounds slightly when dropped from a spoon. Beat the egg whites until stiff. Beat in the remaining acesulfame-K. Fold the gelatin mixture into the stiffly beaten egg whites. Turn into a baked pie shell, if desired. Chill until firm.

Yield: 8 servings   **Exchange:** ½ meat
Each serving contains:
Calories: 46   Fiber: trace
Sodium: 38 mg   Cholesterol: 137 mg

Marion's Lime Pie Filling

Edith's mother had a friend, Marion, who was famous for her desserts. Some were very complicated; some were very, very easy but tasted so wonderful that everyone assumed Marion spent hours making them. This is our version of Marion's pie. Yogurt cheese is made by letting yogurt drip through cheesecloth overnight in the refrigerator.

1 pkg	sugar-free, fat-free lime gelatin	1 pkg
⅓ C	boiling water	90 mL
1¼ C	diet ginger ale	310 mL
1 C	yogurt cheese	250 mL
	whipped topping (optional)	

Dissolve the gelatin in boiling water in a large bowl, stirring with a large spoon. Add the ginger ale. Stir well to combine. Whisk in the yogurt cheese until blended. The mixture will be thin. Freeze for 10 minutes, then spoon into a prepared pie shell until set. Garnish with whipped topping, if desired.

Yield: 8 servings   **Exchange:** free
Each serving contains:
Calories: 19   Fiber: 0
Sodium: 46 mg   Cholesterol: trace

Frozen Raspberry Pie Filling

This is another of Marion's recipes, modified for diabetic use. It tastes very rich and creamy.

1½ C	sugar-free, reduced-fat vanilla ice cream	375 mL
½ C	raspberries	125 mL
1	prepared pie crust	1

Allow the ice cream to soften at room temperature for approximately an hour; add the raspberries and process until smooth in a food processor. Pour into a pie crust shell. Freeze. Allow the pie to soften for a few minutes at room temperature before serving.

Yield: 8 servings   **Exchange:** ½ bread
Each serving contains:
Calories: 41   Fiber: trace
Sodium: 17 mg   Cholesterol: 6 mg

Blueberry Pie Filling

Everyone we know likes blueberry pie. If you can afford the calories and fat exchanges, put this filling between a bottom and top pie crust. If you want a lighter version, put just the filling in an empty pie pan and top it with a fillo crust. This filling is great in a turnover made from fillo dough.

12 oz. bag	frozen blueberries	356 g bag
3 pkts	concentrated acesulfame-K	3 pkts
1½ T	cornstarch dissolved in 2 T (30 mL) water	22 mL
½ t	vanilla extract	2 mL
½ T	lemon juice	7 mL
¼ t	cinnamon	1 mL

Partially defrost the blueberries at room temperature or in a microwave oven for 60 seconds. Combine all the other ingredients in a saucepan, add the blueberries, and heat over medium heat, stirring constantly until the mixture thickens.

Yield: 8 servings　　**Exchange:** ½ fruit
Each serving contains:
Calories: 23　　Fiber: trace
Sodium: 2 mg　　Cholesterol: 0

Pistachio Pineapple Pie Filling

This is very quick to put together and sets up quickly too. It's the type of recipe that makes non-cooks feel successful.

2 pkg	sugar-free pistachio pudding mix	2 pkg
12¼ C	nonfat milk	560 mL
1 t	almond extract	5 mL
1 (8 oz.) can	crushed pineapple (in unsweetened juice)	1 (250 mL) can
1	prepared pie shell	1

Combine the pudding, milk, and almond extract and beat with an electric mixer for one minute. Add the pineapple and its juice and beat for an additional minute. Pour into a prepared pie shell.

Yield: 8 servings　　**Exchange:** 1 bread
Each serving contains:
Calories: 71　　Fiber: trace
Sodium: 366 mg　　Cholesterol: 1.1 mg

Sheer Delight Pie Filling

This dessert is rich and delicious, a special-occasion treat. It's great in a baked graham cracker crust.

1 pkg	sugar-free, fat-free instant pudding	1 pkg
1½ C	nonfat sour cream	310 mL
1 T	rum extract	15 mL
2 T	measures-like-sugar aspartame	30 mL
2 T	nonfat milk	30 mL
1 (8 oz.) can	crushed unsweetened pineapple, in juice, drained	1 (244 g) can
½ C	flaked coconut	125 mL
1	prepared pie shell	1
	banana slices (optional)	
	whipped topping (optional)	

Combine instant pudding, sour cream, rum extract, aspartame, and milk in a medium bowl. Beat the mixture with a wire whisk until blended and smooth, about a minute, then fold in the pineapple and coconut. Spoon everything into a pie shell. Chill for three hours. Before serving, garnish with sliced bananas or your favorite topping (optional).

Yield: 8 servings   **Exchange:** 1 bread + 1 fat + 1 fruit
Each serving contains:
Calories: 181   Fiber: 2 g
Sodium: 227 mg   Cholesterol: 6 mg

Tutti-Frutti Pie

Count the calories and exchanges for the pie crust separately from the filling, depending on which crust you choose. If you choose no crust, just pour the mixture into a pie pan and chill it; you save yourself the trouble of making a crust, and you save calories. This filling is really good and it's quick and easy.

1 env.	plain gelatin	1 env.
2 T	cold water	30 mL
¾ C	nonfat cottage cheese	190 mL
⅓ C	boiling water	90 mL
¼ C	skim milk	60 mL
2 t	vanilla extract	10 mL
½ t	almond extract	2.5 mL
1 t	concentrated aspartame	10 mL
1 lb.	light mixed fruit chunks, drained	450 g

Sprinkle the gelatin over the cold water. Set aside to soften for a few minutes. Meanwhile, put the cottage cheese into a food processor or blender and process for a full 2 minutes to make it very creamy. Add the boiling water to the softened gelatin. Stir until the gelatin is completely dissolved. Add this mixture, milk, extracts, and aspartame to the blender. Blend until the mixture is smooth. Put the canned fruit into the food processor or blender and blend for a few seconds. Pour into a pie crust or into a plain pie pan. Chill until set.

Yield: 8 servings   **Exchange:** ½ bread
Each serving contains:
Calories: 52   Fiber: trace
Sodium: 7 mg   Cholesterol: 2 mg

Luscious Strawberry Pie Filling

If you can find sugar-free, non-fat frozen yogurt, use it as a base for other flavors. By itself it's a little unexciting, but strawberries bring their own special taste.

2 C (1 pint)	frozen whole strawberries with no sugar added	500 mL
1 t	sugar	5 mL
1 t	concentrated aspartame	5 mL
1 t	lemon juice	5 mL
1 C	boiling water	250 mL
1 pkg (.3 oz)	triple berry sugar-free gelatin	1 pkg (8.5 g)
2 t	strawberry extract	10 mL
1 pint	sugar-free vanilla nonfat yogurt	475 mL
1	prepared pie shell	1

Mix the strawberries in a bowl with the sugar, aspartame, and lemon juice. Set aside for approximately an hour. Combine the boiling water and gelatin and stir until completely dissolved. Add the strawberry extract and stir to combine. Add the frozen yogurt and stir until it melts and the mixture is smooth. Freeze for 10 minutes, until the gelatin starts to set. Add the strawberries. Pour into a pie shell of your choice. Refrigerate. Serve when set.

Yield: 8 servings   **Exchange:** 1 fruit
Each serving contains:
Calories: 58   Fiber: trace
Sodium: 63 mg   Cholesterol: 0

Quick Banana Cream Pie Filling

This would be a good project for a cook-in-training. You just can't go wrong. Banana cream pie is traditionally served in a flour-based bottom crust.

1	banana, ripe, sliced thin	1
3 C	skim milk	750 mL
2 pkgs	sugar-free fat-free vanilla pudding	2 pkgs

Place the banana slices in the bottom of the pie shell of your choice. Using an electric mixer, combine the milk and pudding. Pour the mixture over the banana slices. Chill until serving time. Add additional thin slices of banana or whipped topping just before serving, if desired.

Yield: 8 servings   **Exchange:** 1 bread
Each serving contains:
Calories: 70   Fiber: trace
Sodium: 377 mg   Cholesterol: 1.5 mg

Golden Treasure Pie Filling

This is a sugar-free version of an old family favorite. Karin served this on New Year's Day, and no one guessed it was sugar-free.

2 T	cornstarch	30 mL
2 T	water	30 mL
3 pkts	concentrated saccharin	3 pkts
3 pkts	concentrated acesulfame-K	3 pkts
1 T	margarine	15 mL
2 T	sifted flour	30 mL
½ C	nonfat cottage cheese	125 mL
1 t	vanilla extract	5 mL
1	egg white or egg	1
¾ C	nonfat milk	190 mL
2 (8½ oz.) cans	crushed pineapple, packed in juice, undrained	2 (256 g) cans

Combine the cornstarch and water in a small saucepan. Bring to a boil, then cook one minute, stirring constantly. Cool. Stir in the saccharin. In a mixing bowl, blend the acesulfame-K and margarine. Add the flour, cottage cheese, and vanilla. Beat until smooth. Slowly add the egg, and then the milk, to the cheese mixture, beating constantly. Pour the pineapple into a 10-inch (25 cm) crust, if desired, spreading the mixture evenly. Gently pour the cottage cheese over the pineapple, being careful not to disturb the first layer. Bake at

450° F (230°C) for 15 minutes, then reduce the heat to 325°F (160°C) and bake for 45 minutes longer.

Yield: 10 servings   **Exchange:** 1 bread
Each serving contains:
Calories: 68   Fiber: trace
Sodium: 36 mg   Cholesterol: 1.3 mg

Pumpkin-Apple Pie Filling

The first time Karin made this for guests, everyone wanted seconds.

⅓ C	unsweetened apple juice	90 mL
1 T	cornstarch	15 mL
½ t	cinnamon	2 mL
1 t	rum-flavored extract	5 mL
3 C	apples, sliced, cored and peeled	750 mL
	(3 medium or 2 large apples)	
1	egg or equivalent egg substitute	1
¾ C	canned or cooked mashed pumpkin	190 mL
¼ t	ginger	1 mL
½ t	cinnamon	2 mL
⅛ t	cloves	.5 mL
⅓ C	measures-like-sugar aspartame	90 mL
¾ C	evaporated skim milk	190 mL
	sugar-free whipped topping (optional)	

Combine the apple juice, cornstarch, ½ t cinnamon, and rum-flavored extract in a large saucepan. Stir constantly. Bring to a boil. Add the apples. Cook for four minutes over medium heat, stirring constantly.

In a mixing bowl, beat the eggs, then add the pumpkin, ginger, cinnamon, cloves, bulk aspartame, and evaporated skim milk. Stir to blend well.

Turn the apple mixture into a 9-inch (23 cm) pie shell. Spoon the pumpkin mixture over the apple layer, Bake in a preheated 375°F (190°C) oven for 30 minutes until the pumpkin is set and only slightly browned.

Top with sugar-free whipped topping, if desired.

Yield: 8 servings   **Exchange:** 1 bread
Each serving contains:
Calories: 132   Fiber: 3 g
Sodium: 24 mg   Cholesterol: 0

Stove Top Pumpkin Pie Filling

An elegant version of traditional pumpkin pie.

1½ C	cooked or canned pumpkin	375 mL
1½ C	evaporated nonfat milk	375 mL
1 t	cinnamon	5 mL
½ t	ginger	2 mL
⅛ t	cloves	.5 mL
3	eggs, slightly beaten, or equivalent egg substitute	3
1 t	vanilla extract	5 mL
2 t	rum extract	10 mL
20 pkts	concentrated acesulfame-K	20 pkts
1	prepared pie shell	1
	whipped topping (optional)	

Cook the pumpkin, evaporated milk, cinnamon, ginger, cloves, and eggs or egg substitute in the top of a double boiler over hot water, stirring until thick. Cool until the mixture is no longer steaming and add the vanilla and rum extracts and the acesulfame-K.

Beat well, using an electric mixer. Pour into baked pie shell of your choice. Top with sugar-free whipped topping, if desired.

Yield: 8 servings   **Exchange:** ½ milk
Each serving contains:
Calories: 68   Fiber: 2 g
Sodium: 51 mg   Cholesterol: 0 mg

No-Cook Pumpkin Pie Filling

Easy as pie!

1 C	evaporated skim milk	250 mL
1 pkg	unflavored gelatin	1 pkg
1 C	canned pumpkin	250 mL
1 C	nonfat ricotta cheese	250 mL
2 t	pumpkin pie spice	10 mL
1 t	vanilla extract	5 mL
2 T	concentrated aspartame	30 mL
	whipped topping (optional)	

Pour the evaporated milk into a small bowl. Sprinkle the gelatin on it and let the gelatin soften for a few minutes. In a food processor, combine the rest of the ingredients. With a wire whisk, stir the gelatin gently into the evaporated milk until it is dissolved. Add this to the ingredients in the food processor and blend well. Pour into prepared pie crust, if desired. Refrigerate.

If desired, garnish each slice with 2 T (30 mL) of low-fat, low-sugar whipped topping.

Yield: 8 servings   **Exchange:** ½ milk
    Each serving contains:
    Calories: 63   Fiber: 1.5 g
    Sodium: 22 mg   Cholesterol: 2.5 mg

Quick Pumpkin Pie Filling

Using convenience foods, such as pudding mixes, is great for busy cooks. The egg substitute, canned pumpkin, and nonfat milk add protein and fiber.

½ C	egg substitute or 2 eggs	125 mL
1 C	canned pumpkin	250 mL
1½ C	nonfat milk	375 mL
1 t	pumpkin pie spice	5 mL
1 t	vanilla extract	5 mL
1 t	concentrated aspartame	5 mL
1 (1 oz.) pkg	fat-free sugar-free vanilla-pudding mix	1 (28 g) pkg
1 (1 oz.) pkg	fat-free sugar-free butterscotch-pudding mix	1 (28 g) pkg

Use an electric mixer to combine all ingredients. Mix well, then pour into a prepared pie shell. Refrigerate until served.

Yield: 8 servings   **Exchange:** 1 bread
    Each serving contains:
    Calories: 63   Fiber: 1 g
    Sodium: 387 mg   Cholesterol: trace

Frozen Chocolate Pie Filling

This is a delightful dessert for a summer evening. Try the Graham Cracker Crust recipe (page 73) or use your choice of crust.

2 C	sugar-free, reduced-fat chocolate ice cream	500 mL
¾ C	diet double fudge soda	90 mL
¼ t	chocolate extract	1 mL
1 t	bulk aspartame	5 mL
¼ C	nonfat ricotta cheese	60 mL
1 t	imitation brandy flavor	5 mL

Allow the ice cream to soften at room temperature for approximately an hour. Meanwhile, combine the next four ingredients with a wire whisk to make a glaze. Pour into a prebaked graham cracker crust. Freeze. Process the ricotta cheese and brandy flavoring in a food processor until smooth, about a minute. Add the softened ice cream and process until very smooth. Pour into a prepared pie crust.

Yield: 8 servings　　**Exchange:** ½ bread
Each serving contains:
Calories: 56　　Fiber: trace
Sodium: 28 mg　　Cholesterol: 8 mg

Creamy Mocha Pie Filling

This is an easy pie to assemble; we didn't find anyone who didn't like it. It's good in a graham cracker crust.

1 pkg	unflavored gelatin	1 pkg
½ C	water	125 mL
1 C	skim milk	250 mL
¾ C	fat-free ricotta cheese	190 mL
⅓ C	unsweetened cocoa powder	60 mL
1 t	instant coffee granules dissolved in 1 C (250 mL) boiling water	5 mL
2 t	chocolate extract	10 mL
10 pkts	aspartame	10 pkts
	prepared pie (see pages 70–75)	

Combine the gelatin and water in a saucepan; after a few minutes, heat until the gelatin is dissolved. In a blender or food processor, combine the remaining ingredients. Add the dissolved gelatin and blend. Pour into a prepared pie shell and refrigerate.

Yield: 8 servings   **Exchange:** ½ milk
Each serving contains:
Calories: 33   Fiber: trace
Sodium: 32 mg   Cholesterol: 2.4 mg

Turnovers

A turnover is a piece of pastry wrapped around a filling, usually fruit-based. When you use fillo dough for the pastry, you get a turnover with a relatively low cost in calories and exchanges, depending of course on the filling you choose. One sheet of fillo dough makes a large turnover. Half would be considered a serving. Fillo dough with fruit filling in it is best eaten on the day it is baked.

| 4 sheets | fillo dough | 4 sheets |
| 1 C | filling | 250 mL |

Follow the general directions for fillo dough. Spread out one large sheet, coat with butter-flavored non-stick vegetable cooking spray. Fold the dough into thirds the long way. Spray again. Put ¼ C (60 mL) filling on the dough about 2 inches (5 cm) from the bottom. Using your fingers, fold the dough up and over the filling; then press down gently. Fold this filled section up towards the plain dough. Fold it up again, as if you were folding a flag. Continue until all the dough has been folded up over the filling. Use your fingers to be sure it is sealed at the edges. Spray the dough again. Put the turnover on a cookie sheet that has been sprayed with non-stick vegetable cooking spray. Repeat with the other three turnovers, or as many as you want. Bake in a preheated 375°F (190°C) oven for 10 minutes.

Yield: 4 turnovers (filling counted separately) **Exchange:** 1 bread
Each one contains:
Calories: 72   Fiber: trace
Sodium: 120 mg   Cholesterol: 0

Apple Turnovers

Need something to serve in a pinch? These turnovers can be made in only 10 minutes and are quite tasty.

2 slices	bread (crust removed)	2 slices
1	apple, peeled, cored and sliced thin	1
1 t	lemon juice	5 mL
¼ t	cinnamon	1 mL
1 pkt	concentrated acesulfame-K	1 pkt

Roll the bread thin with a rolling pin. Microwave the other ingredients until the apple is tender. The length of time will depend on the type of apple and the power of the oven. I start with 10 seconds on medium and adjust from there. The key is, you don't want the apple mushy. Place half the mixture on each piece of bread. Fold the bread diagonally to form a triangle. Moisten the edges of the bread and press the sides of the turnover together with fork. Lightly spray both sides with vegetable cooking spray. Place on a cookie sheet coated with non-stick vegetable cooking spray. Bake at 425°F (220°C) for about 7 minutes or until brown.

Yield: 2 turnovers   **Exchange:** 1 bread + ½ fruit
Each turnover contains:
Calories: 95   Fiber: 2 g
Sodium: 102 mg   Cholesterol: 1 mg

CHAPTER SIX

Fruits

Many people with diabetes save a fruit to have as their dessert. You don't need a cookbook for this. In this chapter we offer fancier desserts that are basically fruits. Taking a fruit exchange and turning it into an attractive healthy dessert makes sense for everyone in the family.

Sweet 'n Sour Strawberries

Surprisingly flavorful and so easy! Serve in fancy glasses.

2 C	fresh or frozen strawberries with no sugar added	500 mL
3 pkts	concentrated acesulfame-K	3 pkts
2 T	balsamic vinegar	30 mL

Slice the strawberries in half. Sprinkle them with acesulfame-K and vinegar. Stir to combine. This is best served chilled.

> **Yield:** 4 servings   **Exchange:** free
> **Each serving contains:**
> Calories: 24   Fiber: 2 g
> Sodium: trace   Cholesterol: 0

Zesty Strawberries

Adding black pepper to strawberries is unusual but very tasty. Try it! You'll like it.

2 C	fresh strawberries, sliced	500 mL
1½ t	concentrated aspartame	7 mL
½ t	cracked black pepper	2 mL
½ t	brandy extract	2 mL
2 T	diet cream soda	30 mL

Stir all the ingredients together and chill before serving. Zesty Strawberries can be served plain or over a frozen ice cream substitute.

> **Yield:** 8 servings   **Exchange:** free
> **Each serving contains:**
> Calories: 11   Fiber: trace
> Sodium: trace   Cholesterol: 0

Cool Strawberry Fluff

A light, frothy dessert, Cool Strawberry Fluff will melt in your mouth. Serve it after a heavy meal for the best effect.

10 oz. (1¼ C)	fresh or frozen strawberries sliced, no sugar added	300 g (310 mL)
2 env. (2 T)	unflavored gelatin	2 env. (30 mL)
1 C	coarsely crushed ice	250 mL

Put ½ C (125 mL) strawberries into a blender and blend them for about 5 seconds. Pour them into a small saucepan and heat over low heat until they begin to boil, then transfer them back into the blender. Sprinkle the gelatin over the hot strawberries, cover, and blend for about 30 seconds more. Add the crushed ice and blend at the lowest speed for 20 seconds. Put the remaining strawberries in a bowl, add the pureed mixture, and mix together for about 30 seconds. Pour into individual dishes or a serving bowl. Chill.

Yield: 4 servings **Exchange:** free
Each serving contains:
Calories: 26 calories   Fiber: trace
Sodium: 3 mg   Cholesterol: 0

Fresh Strawberry-Melon Medley

This was a favorite among our friends. They loved the festive way it looked and tasted and couldn't believe how simple it was to prepare!

10 oz.	defrosted sliced strawberries, no sugar added	300 g
1½ C	water	375 mL
½	stick cinnamon	½
3 T	cornstarch	45 mL
¼ C	cold water	60 mL
3 pkts	concentrated acesulfame-K	3 pkts
2 C	fresh strawberries, quartered	500 mL
2 C	honeydew melon balls (fresh or frozen)	500 mL

In a saucepan combine the thawed strawberries, 1½ C (375 mL) water, and cinnamon; bring to a boil, then simmer for five minutes. Puree in a blender or food processor. In another bowl, blend the cornstarch, ¼ C (60 mL) cold water, and acesulfame-K. Stir into the puree. Bring to a boil, stirring constantly, then simmer for one minute. Pour into a bowl; place a piece of wax paper on the surface; let cool, then refrigerate.

Before serving, remove the wax paper. Beat the puree until fluffy. Fold in the fresh strawberries and melon balls, reserving a few of each for the garnish. Spoon into parfait glasses; top with the reserved strawberries and melon balls.

Yield: 6 servings   Exchange: 1½ fruit
Each serving contains:
Calories: 104   Fiber: 3 g
Sodium: 18 mg   Cholesterol: 0

Double Melon Dessert

If you don't have a melon ball scoop, dice 3 C melon or use frozen melon. Annette thinks this is perfect for an afternoon snack on a summer day or as a sorbet after a fancy meal.

2	cantaloupes (or 1 large honeydew melon)	2
2 pkgs	sugar-free orange-flavored gelatin	2 pkgs
1	orange	1

Scoop out enough melon balls to equal 3 C (750 mL). Chill. Using a spoon, scrape out the remainder of the melon. Puree. Measure the pureed melon. Add water, if needed, to make 4 C. Pour into a saucepan. Heat until steaming. Remove from the heat, add gelatin, and stir until the gelatin is dissolved. Pour into six custard cups and chill until firm. Garnish each serving with ½ C (125 mL) of melon balls and orange slices.

Yield: 6 servings   Exchange: 1 bread
Each serving contains:
Calories: 88   Fiber: 2 g
Sodium: 83 mg   Cholesterol: 0

Applesauce

Unsweetened applesauce in a glass jar is about as convenient as a diabetic dessert can be. Edith's diabetic friend Bob suggested putting applesauce in the cookbook because he always likes the way Edith dresses it up with aspartame and cinnamon. We didn't think that just adding aspartame and cinnamon to commercial applesauce was actually a recipe! But maybe the advice on sweet sprinkles will give you some good ideas.

Sweet Sprinkles

Mix an artificial sweetener of your choice with other spices. Put the mixture into a clean salt shaker or other small shaker container. Here are some combinations our tasters liked: equal parts of aspartame and cinnamon; aspartame and cardamom; aspartame and pumpkin pie spice.

Baked Apples

Baked apples are easy to make, and the apple juice makes them especially moist. Just put them in the oven before you start the rest of your dinner preparations. The smell coming from the oven will tantalize you.

4	medium baking apples	4
1 t	fructose	5 mL
⅓ C	canned crushed pineapple, packed in juice, drained	90 mL
2 T	raisins (optional)	30 mL
¼ t	cinnamon	1 mL
2–4 C	unsweetened apple juice	500 mL–1 L

Peel the top of each apple. Use a sharp knife to remove the core, but leave the bottom intact so the hollow can be filled. Cut a thin slice from the bottom, if necessary, so the apple stands upright. In a small bowl, combine the fructose, pineapple, raisins, and cinnamon. Spoon the mixture equally into each apple hollow. Place the apples in a shallow baking dish. Surround the apples with apple juice to a depth of about ½ inch (1.25 cm). Bake in a preheated 350°F (180°C) oven for about an hour. The apples should be tender, but not mushy. Serve warm, at room temperature, or chilled and garnish with sugar-free nonfat whipped topping just before serving.

Yield: 4 servings   **Exchange:** 2 fruits
Each serving contains:
Calories: 110   Fiber: 4 g
Sodium: 8   Cholesterol: 0

Apple Crisp

An apple crisp baking fills a home with the most wonderful aroma, and you get to eat the apple too!

4 C	apples, sliced	1 L
¼ C	water	60 mL
1 T	molasses	15 mL
3 pkts	concentrated acesulfame-K	3 pkts
1 T	lemon juice	15 mL
1 t	cinnamon	5 mL
¼ t	cloves	1 mL
¾ C	oatmeal	190 mL
2 t	margarine or butter	10 mL
2 pkts	concentrated acesulfame-K	2 pkts

Combine the apples, water, molasses, acesulfame-K, lemon juice, cinnamon, and cloves. Mix well. Arrange the apple mixture in an 8-inch (20 cm) square baking dish coated with non-stick cooking spray. Combine the remaining ingredients and sprinkle the mixture over the apples. Bake at 375°F (190°C) for 30 minutes or until the apples are tender and the topping is lightly browned.

Yield: 8 servings   **Exchange:** 1 bread
Each serving contains:
Calories: 84   Fiber: 2 g
Sodium: 12 mg   Cholesterol: 0

Betty-Style Apples

Apple Betty is a casserole of apples and bread crumbs. It's rich and delicious.

1½ C	fresh bread crumbs	375 mL
¼ C	melted margarine or butter	60 mL
4 pkts	concentrated acesulfame-K	4 pkts
¼ t	nutmeg	1 mL
¼ t	cinnamon	1 mL
3	medium apples, pared, cored, and sliced thin	3
1½ t	lemon juice	7 mL
3 T	water	45 mL
1 pkt	concentrated acesulfame-K	1 pkt

Toss the bread crumbs and margarine. In a small bowl, combine the four packets of acesulfame-K and the nutmeg and cinnamon. In a 1-quart (1 liter) casserole arrange one-third of the crumbs. On top of the crumbs arrange one-third of the apples. Sprinkle the apples with one-third of the cinnamon mixture. Add another layer of crumbs, apples. Do this again. Top with the remaining crumbs. Mix together the lemon juice, water, and one packet of acesulfame-K. Drizzle over the top layer of crumbs. Cover and bake in a preheated 350°F (180°C) oven for 15 minutes, then uncover and bake 30 minutes longer. Serve warm or cold.

Yield: 8 servings   **Exchanges:** 1 fat + ½ bread + ½ fruit
Each serving contains:
Calories: 117   Fiber: 2 g
Sodium: 83 mg   Cholesterol: 0

Apple Dessert

Karin loves this recipe because it's fast and easy to make with ingredients that are usually on hand. Shake on a little nutmeg and cinnamon if you like.

1 C	unsweetened applesauce	250 mL
½ T	lemon juice	7 mL
½ t	vanilla extract	2 mL
1 env.	gelatin	1 env.
¼ C	cold water	60 mL
½ C	hot water	60 mL

Mix together the applesauce, lemon juice, and vanilla extract. Soften the gelatin in cold water for five minutes. Add the hot water and stir until it is dissolved. Then add the water and gelatin to the applesauce mixture. Refrigerate the mixture. When it begins to stiffen, beat it until light.

Yield: 6 servings   **Exchange:** free
Each serving contains:
Calories: 22   Fiber: trace
Sodium: 2 mg   Cholesterol: 0

Nectarine Crisp

Nectarines are available fresh most of the year and are great to cook with.

1 C	rolled oats	250 mL
¼ C	apple juice concentrate	60 mL
1 t	cornstarch	5 mL
4	nectarines, peeled and sliced thin	4
3 T	flour	45 mL
1½ t	cinnamon	7 mL
¼ t	nutmeg	1 mL
3 pkts	acesulfame-K	3 pkts
2 T	diet pancake syrup, sugar-free	30 mL
2 T	nonfat sour cream	30 mL

Spread the rolled oats flat in a large pan. Bake in a preheated 325°F (160°C) oven for 10 minutes. Remove from the oven and set aside. Meanwhile, in a saucepan stir together the apple juice concentrate and cornstarch and cook over medium heat until thickened, stirring constantly. Spread the nectarine slices evenly over the bottom of a small ovenproof dish that has been coated with non-stick cooking spray. Pour the apple juice-cornstarch mixture over the slices. Then combine the flour, cinnamon, nutmeg, and acesulfame-K with the oatmeal. Add the pancake syrup and sour cream to the flour-oatmeal and stir to combine. Crumble this mixture over the nectarines. Bake in a preheated 325°F (160°C) oven for 45 minutes.

Yield: 6 servings   **Exchange:** 1 bread + ½ fruit
Each serving contains:
Calories: 140   Fiber: 3 g
Sodium: 16 mg   Cholesterol: trace

Nectarine Puree

Use fresh, sweet nectarines in season for the best result.

3	nectarines	3
2 t	lemon juice	10 mL
2 t	concentrated aspartame	10 mL

Drop the nectarines into a large pan of boiling water. Shut off the heat. Let stand for one minute to loosen the skins. Drain the hot water; then pour cold water over the fruit and slip off their skins. Place the nectarines in a food processor or blender with the lemon juice and aspartame. The amount of aspartame will vary, depending on the tartness of the fruit. Puree. Spoon into glass dessert dishes.

Yield: 3 servings   **Exchange:** 1 fruit
Each serving contains:
Calories: 68   Fiber: 3 g
Sodium: trace   Cholesterol: 0

Browned Bananas

You can't imagine how satisfying a simple broiled banana can be until you've tried this recipe.

1	banana, peeled	1

Slice the banana in half the long way. Place it on a broiler pan that has been coated with non-stick cooking spray. Place the pan under a preheated broiler a few inches from the heat. Watch it carefully and remove the tray from the oven as the banana becomes browned and bubbly. Serve hot. No garnish is necessary, but some people like to serve it with a small amount of sugar-free frozen nonfat vanilla yogurt.

Yield: 2 servings   **Exchange:** 1 fruit
Each serving contains:
Calories: 53   Fiber: 1 g
Sodium: trace   Cholesterol: 0

Elegant Blueberry Dessert

A very fancy way to serve a dessert that is basically just fruit.

½ C	nonfat milk	125 mL
2 t	cornstarch	10 mL
2 T	orange liqueur (optional)	30 mL
2 pkts	concentrated acesulfame-K	2 pkts
2 t	vanilla extract	10 mL
1 t	concentrated aspartame-K	5 mL
1	egg white	1
pinch	cream of tartar	pinch
2 C	blueberries (fresh or frozen without sugar and defrosted)	500 mL

Stir together the milk, cornstarch, liqueur if desired, and acesulfame-K in a medium saucepan. Use a wire whisk to be sure the cornstarch is dissolved. Bring to a boil and reduce the heat to a simmer, stirring constantly. Turn off the heat and stir in the vanilla extract and aspartame.

In a separate bowl, beat the egg white until it holds its peaks, add the cream of tartar, and continue beating until the white is stiff. Fold it into the milk-cornstarch mixture. Then stir in the blueberries. Pour the mixture into four fancy glasses, such as wine glasses. Chill.

Yield: 4 servings   **Exchange:** 1 bread
Each serving contains:
Calories: 60   Fiber: 2 g
Sodium: 33 mg   Cholesterol: trace

Watermelon Pudding

This is a great way to serve the watermelon left over after a picnic. At Karin's house in the summer there are always crowds of people (especially at mealtimes), but no matter what size watermelon, there's always some left over. This recipe is a great way to use it up.

3 C	pureed watermelon	750 mL
1 T	lemon juice	15 mL
1 env.	unflavored gelatin	1 env.
1 pkg	strawberry-flavored gelatin dessert	1 pkg
¾ lb.	nonfat cottage cheese	340 g

In a saucepan, combine the watermelon puree, lemon juice, and unflavored gelatin. Let it stand for five minutes or so to soften. Heat gently until the gelatin dissolves. Remove from the heat and stir in the strawberry-flavored gelatin. Stir until the mixture is smooth and the gelatin is dissolved. Pour half the mixture into six custard cups coated with non-stick cooking spray. Chill until set. Pour the remainder into a blender or food processor. Add the cottage cheese and blend. Pour the blended cheese on top of the first mixture. Chill until firm.

Serve in cups or unmould onto dessert plates. (To unmould custard cups, run a hot knife around the inside of each cup, dip the knife into a pan of hot water for a few seconds. Put a plate over the top of the cup. Invert, shake onto the plate.)

Yield: 6 servings　　　　**Exchange:** 1 fruit
Each serving contains:
Calories: 85　　　　　　　Fiber: 1.6 g
Sodium: 7 mg　　　　　　Cholesterol: 0

Poached Pears and Raspberries

When you find out how easy this fabulous recipe is, you'll stop being so impressed with poached pear desserts at the most chic restaurants.

6	medium pears	6
1 pkt	concentrated acesulfame-K, or 1 T (15 mL) sugar	1 pkt
¼ C	water	60 mL
1-inch	piece of vanilla bean, slit	2.5 cm
2 C	raspberries, fresh or frozen, unsweetened	500 mL
2 T	fruit-only jam (seedless raspberry is a good choice)	30 mL

Peel, core, and halve the pears. Combine the acesulfame or sugar and water in a saucepan and bring to a boil. Reduce the heat to low and add the vanilla bean and pear halves. Cover. Simmer for 5 minutes or so, until the pears are fork-tender. Cool. Drain. In a small bowl, gently toss the raspberries and jelly. Put two pear halves on each serving plate. Mound the raspberries on top of the pears.

Yield: 6 servings　　　　**Exchange:** 2 fruits
Each serving contains:
Calories: 168　　　　　　Fiber: 7 g
Sodium: 0　　　　　　　　Cholesterol: 0

Pears à la Crème

When you see pears in the grocery store, think of this recipe and the fabulous dessert it makes.

2	large firm pears, peeled, cored	2
1 pkt	concentrated acesulfame-K, or 1 T (15 mL) sugar	15 mL
¼ C	unsweetened pineapple juice	60 mL
1 C	sugar-free whipped topping	250 mL
4 pkts	concentrated aspartame	4 pkts

Cut the pears into large chunks. Combine the pears, acesulfame-K, and pineapple juice. Bring to a boil, stirring constantly until the sugar dissolves. Cover, reduce heat, and cook until the fruit is fork-tender. The time will vary depending on the hardness of the fruit. This step may be very short. Uncover, increase the heat, and cook until the juices thicken. Cool until serving time. Fold in the topping and aspartame just before serving.

Yield: 6 servings   **Exchange:** 1 fruit
Each serving contains:
Calories: 52   Fiber: 1.6 g
Sodium: 7 mg   Cholesterol: 0

Ambrosia

When oranges are sweet and juicy, ambrosia can be as delectable as any elaborate dessert.

2	oranges, peeled with any bitter white skin removed	2
2 t	measures-like-sugar aspartame	10 mL
2	bananas, peeled	2
¼ C	shredded coconut (optional)	125 mL

Slice the oranges and bananas thin. Place a layer of orange slices in the bottom of a serving bowl. Sprinkle with some of the aspartame. Place a layer of bananas over the oranges, then a layer of coconut. Make many layers of fruit, ending with a layer of coconut. Cover with plastic wrap; refrigerate for at least an hour before serving.

Yield: 4 servings   **Exchange:** 1½ fruit
Each serving contains:
Calories: 84   Fiber: 3 g
Sodium: trace   Cholesterol: 0

Grapefruit Meringue

Grapefruit isn't just for breakfast anymore! Baked with a crown of meringue, the grapefruit becomes sweet and dramatic.

2	medium grapefruit	2
3	egg whites	3
3 pkts	concentrated acesulfame-K	3 pkts

Cut the grapefruit in half; snip the center core from each half, then cut around all sections, and arrange the halves in a shallow baking dish lined with aluminum foil. Beat the egg whites until they are stiff enough to hold their shape; gradually add the acesulfame-K, beating until they are stiff. Pile some of meringue mixture on top of each grapefruit half. Bake for 15 minutes in a 375°F (190°C) oven.

Yield: 4 servings   **Exchange:** 1 fruit
Each serving contains:
Calories: 50   Fiber: trace
Sodium: 38 mg   Cholesterol: 0

Mixed Berry Smoothie

Many grocery stores sell unsweetened fruits in collections. The combination of raspberries, strawberries, and blueberries is a natural for easy desserts.

1 (12 oz.) can	evaporated nonfat milk	1 (354 mL) can
1 T	cornstarch	15 mL
3 pkts	concentrated acesulfame-K	3 pkts
1 t	almond extract	5 mL
1 t	concentrated aspartame	5 mL
1 (12 oz.) bag	frozen mixed berries	1 (340 g) bag
2 C	nonfat yogurt, no sugar added (plain or vanilla)	500 mL

Combine the first three ingredients and stir them together in a saucepan. Heat just to the boil, then reduce the heat and simmer for 5 minutes or until the sauce thickens. Stir constantly with a wire whisk. Turn off the heat; stir in the almond extract, aspartame, and berries. Let cool and then fold in the yogurt.

Yield: 8 servings   **Exchange:** 1 milk
Each serving contains:
Calories: 99   Fiber: 1 g
Sodium: 93 mg   Cholesterol: 0

Elegant Fruit with Almonds

This really is an elegant dessert that you can put together with cans from your shelf. Leave the almonds out if you don't need the fat.

20 oz.	pineapple chunks, packed in juice (reserve the juice)	600 g
16 oz.	sliced peaches, fresh or canned, unsweetened	480 g
1 T	safflower oil	15 mL
4 T	slivered almonds	60 mL
1 T	lemon juice	15 mL
5 T	unsweetened pineapple juice (from the can of pineapples)	75 mL

Drain the canned fruits and save the juice. Drop the fruit into a serving bowl and refrigerate. Heat the oil in a small frying pan; add the almonds and cook gently, stirring until they are lightly browned. Remove from the heat and let cool. Add the lemon juice and pineapple juice to the almonds and stir; toss over fruit. Refrigerate until serving time. This is best served chilled.

Yield: 6 servings   **Exchange:** 1 fruit + 1 fat + ½ bread
Each serving contains:
Calories: 153   Fiber: 2 g
Sodium: 6 mg   Cholesterol: 0

Four-Fruit Compote

Oranges, cantaloupe, grapes, and pears are the four fruits we used in this compote. They blend together very well to make an attractive and succulent dessert.

1	large orange	1
1	small cantaloupe	1
½ lb.	seedless grapes	225 g
3	ripe pears	3
½ C	water	125 mL
3 T	lemon juice	45 mL
3 pkts	concentrated acesulfame-K	3 pkts
¼ t	mace	1 mL
2 T	rum (optional)	30 mL

Cut the orange into segments, remove the membrane, and put the segments into a large bowl. Cut the cantaloupe into wedges about 2 inches (5 cm) wide. Remove the seeds and skin. Cut the wedges into large cubes. Add the cubes and the stemmed grapes to the oranges. Cut the pears into quarters, remove the cores, then cut the pears into large cubes. Sprinkle them with lemon juice and add them to the fruit mixture.

Mix together the water, lemon juice, acesulfame-K, and mace. Add the rum, if desired. Cover; refrigerate for an hour or more before serving.

Yield: 8 servings   **Exchange:** 1 fruit
Each serving contains:
Calories: 76   Fiber: 3 g
Sodium: 8 mg   Cholesterol: 0

Peaches and Black Cherries

Take advantage of succulent, fresh, ripe peaches when they are in season and make this dramatic combination.

6	peaches	6
1 T	sugar or 1 pkt. concentrated acesulfame-K	15 mL
⅓ C	water	60 mL
12	black cherries	12
¾ C	sugar-free soda (black cherry or raspberry is a good choice)	190 mL

Dip the peaches one at a time in a pan of boiling water. Plunge them into cold water and slip off the skins. Discard the water. Mix the sugar or acesulfame-K and ⅓ C water in a saucepan large enough to hold all six peaches. Bring the sugar and water to boiling point. Cook gently and add the peaches. Continue to cook gently for 5 more minutes or so. Cool the peaches and their liquid. Before serving, drain the peaches, saving the liquid. Slice the peaches into dessert glasses. Add the cherries. Mix the soda and peach juice together and pour it over the fruit.

Yield: 6 servings   **Exchange:** ½ fruit
Each serving contains:
Calories: 43   Fiber: 1 g
Sodium: 5 mg   Cholesterol: 0

CHAPTER SEVEN

Puddings and Gelatins

"Mom" foods such as rice pudding and custard remind many of us of our childhood. We have taken classic pudding recipes and adapted them to diabetic cooking. Before baking puddings in the oven, put them into separate little "custard" dishes and bake them in a hot water bath. The separate little dishes cook faster and the hot water bath also helps prevent the pudding from developing a rubbery texture, an unfortunate tendency of egg whites and egg substitutes. Low-fat dishes in general benefit from a hot water bath to bake in.

We also offer many gelatin recipes. The new packaged gelatins with aspartame make almost instant desserts. Some people like to make up two different flavors of gelatin in contrasting colors in large flat pans. Then after the gelatin has set, it can be cut into cubes and the cubes combined in a fancy glass. You can alternate red and green gelatin cubes at Christmas. Or combine red and blue cubes with a little whipped topping for the Fourth of July.

The recipes we present use plain, unflavored gelatin, which can yield some lovely desserts. Many are close to being free in terms of diabetic exchanges. Once people get used to using plain gelatin, they often come to prefer it to the artificially colored and flavored varieties.

Grape-Nuts Pudding I

This classic dessert is like the ones delicatessens and diners offer for dessert.

2 C	skim milk	500 mL
½ C	egg substitute	125 mL
4 pkts	concentrated acesulfame-K	4 pkts
pinch	salt (optional)	pinch
1 t	vanilla extract	5 mL
1 t	almond extract	5 mL
½ t	cinnamon	2.5 mL
⅓ C	Grape-Nuts cereal	90 mL
¼ C	golden raisins	60 mL

Heat the milk over hot water in the top of a double boiler. In a bowl, whisk together the egg substitute, acesulfame-K, salt, extracts, and spices. Pour the hot milk slowly over the egg mixture, stirring constantly with a wire whisk. Stir in the Grape-Nuts and raisins. Pour the mixture into eight ovenproof custard cups that have been coated with non-stick vegetable cooking spray.

Place these in a large pan. Pour hot water into the pan to the top of the outside of the custard cups. Place this pan in a preheated 350°F (180°C) oven and bake about an hour. A knife inserted in the center of each pudding should come out clean. Serve warm or chilled.

Yield: 8 servings   **Exchange:** 1 milk
  Each serving contains:
  Calories: 65   Fiber: trace
  Sodium: 94 mg   Cholesterol: 1 mg

Grape-Nuts Pudding II

This is a light and airy sort of Grape-Nuts pudding.

4	egg whites	4
½ C	nonfat sour cream	125 mL
12 pkts	concentrated acesulfame-K	12 pkts
1 T	sugar	15 mL
2 t	grated lemon peel	15 mL
½ C	egg substitute	125 mL
2 C	skim milk	500 mL
½ C	Grape-Nuts cereal	125 mL
⅓ C	flour	90 mL
¼ C	fresh lemon juice	60 mL
sprinkling	nutmeg	sprinkling

Use an electric mixer to beat the egg whites until stiff peaks form. Set them aside. Then use the electric mixer to combine the sour cream with the acesulfame-K, sugar, and lemon peel. Beat until fluffy. Beat in the egg substitute. Then add the milk, cereal, flour, and lemon juice. Stir in a small amount of beaten egg whites to lighten the mixture. Then use a rubber spatula to fold in the remaining egg whites. Pour the mixture into a large ovenproof baking dish that has been coated with non-stick cooking spray and sprinkled with nutmeg. Place this dish in a larger pan filled with hot water. Bake in a preheated 350°F (180°C) oven for 1¼ hours.

Yield: 16 servings   **Exchange:** ½ milk
  Each serving contains:
  Calories: 51   Fiber: trace
  Sodium: 77 mg   Cholesterol: 1.5 mg

Rice Pudding

Like Grandmom used to make but without the fat and sugar. Grandmom would love it!

2 C	skim milk	500 mL
½ C	egg substitute	125 mL
3 pkts	concentrated acesulfame-K	3 pkts
pinch	salt (optional)	pinch
1 T	vanilla extract	30 mL
½ t	cinnamon	2 mL
¾ C	cooked rice	180 mL
¼ C	raisins	60 mL
sprinkling	nutmeg	sprinkling

Heat the milk over hot water in the top of a double boiler. Whisk together the egg substitute, acesulfame-K, and seasonings in a bowl. Pour the hot milk slowly over the egg mixture, stirring with a wire whisk. Stir in the rice and raisins. Pour into eight ovenproof custard cups that have been coated with non-stick cooking spray. Sprinkle the top of each with nutmeg. Place them in a large pan with hot water almost to the top of the custard cups. Place the pan in a preheated 350°F (180°C) oven and bake for about an hour. A knife inserted into the center of each pudding should come out clean. Serve hot or chilled.

Yield: 8 servings   **Exchange:** 1 bread
Each serving contains:
Calories: 73   Fiber: trace
Sodium: 66 mg   Cholesterol: 1 mg

Bread Pudding

This bread pudding is low in calories and exchanges but still has the genuine bread-pudding taste.

½ loaf	"light" sourdough bread	½ loaf
1 (12 oz.) can	evaporated skim milk	1 (375 mL) can
½ C	unsweetened applesauce	125 mL
1 t	vanilla extract	5 mL
½ C	skim milk	125 mL
8 pkts	acesulfame-K	8 pkts
⅓ C	raisins	90 mL
½ t	cinnamon	2 mL
4	egg whites	4

Cut the bread slices into cubes; place them on a cookie sheet coated with non-stick cooking spray. Place the tray in a preheated 350°F (180°C) oven for 10 minutes. Combine all the other ingredients and add the bread. Toss well and place in an ovenproof baking dish that has been sprayed with non-stick vegetable cooking spray. Place this baking dish in a large pan of water filled nearly to the top of the baking dish, and place the pan in a preheated 350°F (180°C) oven. Bake for 40 minutes. Serve hot or cold.

Yield: 8 servings   **Exchange:** 1½ breads
Each serving contains:
Calories: 109   Fiber: 4 g
Sodium: 128 mg   Cholesterol: trace

Baked Custard

Custard is a real "mom" food. There is something comforting about its smooth richness. This recipe uses skim milk and egg substitute, so it's much lower in fat and calories than the old-fashioned kind.

1 (12 oz.) can	evaporated skim milk	1 (375 mL) can
2 pkts	acesulfame-K	2 pkts
1 t	sugar	5 mL
1 t	lemon peel	5 mL
1 t	margarine or butter	5 mL
¼ C	egg substitute	60 mL
1 t	vanilla extract	5 mL
sprinkling	nutmeg (optional)	sprinkling

Heat the milk over hot water in the top of a double boiler. Add the acesulfame-K, sugar, lemon peel, and margarine and whisk together for a few minutes. In a separate bowl, use an electric mixer to beat the egg substitute for a few minutes until foamy and light. Add a little hot milk mixture to the beaten egg substitute and beat. Gradually pour in the rest of the hot milk and beat constantly. Add the vanilla extract and heat briefly. Pour into small ovenproof custard dishes that have been coated with non-stick cooking spray. If desired, sprinkle the top with nutmeg. Place the small cups in a larger pan of hot water. Bake in a preheated 325°F (160°C) oven for approximately 40 minutes. A knife inserted in the center should come out clean. Chill before serving.

Yield: 4 servings   **Exchange:** 1 milk
Each serving contains:
Calories: 97   Fiber: trace
Sodium: 153 mg   Cholesterol: 0

Raspberry Pudding

Raspberries are a natural for low-fat, low-sugar cooking because they add such a nice flavor. They also help to cover up any taste of artificial sweeteners.

½	loaf "light" sourdough bread	½
1 (12 oz.)	can evaporated skim milk	1 (354 mL)
½ C	unsweetened applesauce	125 mL
1 t	vanilla extract	5 mL
½ C	skim milk	125 mL
1 T	sugar	15 mL
8 pkts	concentrated acesulfame-K	8 pkts
½ C	egg substitute	125 mL
½ C	raspberries	125 mL

Cut the bread into large cubes. Put the cubes into an ovenproof baking dish that has been coated with non-stick cooking spray. Use a food processor to combine the other ingredients; pour the mixture over the cubes. Let it sit a few minutes so the bread soaks in some of the wet mixture. Place the baking dish in a large pan of hot water nearly to the top of the baking dish. Bake in a preheated 350°F (180°C) oven for 35 minutes. Serve hot or cold.

Yield: 8 servings　　**Exchange:** 1½ breads
Each serving contains:
Calories: 111　　Fiber: 4 g
Sodium: 162 mg　　Cholesterol: trace

Indian Pudding

As good as any restaurant dessert. If you require a topping, try one-quarter cup of frozen, no-sugar-added, low-fat or nonfat vanilla yogurt.

3½ C	skim milk	875 mL
½ C	cornmeal	125 mL
2 T	molasses	30 mL
¼ C	diet pancake syrup (sugar-free and fructose-free if either elevates *your* blood sugar)	125 mL
2 pkts	concentrated acesulfame-K	2 pkts
2 t	margarine or butter	10 mL
1 t	vanilla extract	5 mL
1 t	cinnamon	5 mL
1 t	ginger	5 mL
½ t	nutmeg	2 mL
pinch	salt (optional)	pinch

| ⅛ t | baking soda | 0.5 mL |
| ¾ C | egg substitute | 190 mL |

Heat 2½ C (625 mL) of milk in a saucepan; bring to a boil. While this is heating, combine ½ C (125 mL) milk and the cornmeal with a wire whisk. When the milk boils, pour in the cornmeal-milk mixture and cook over medium heat. Stir with a wire whisk and cook for approximately 10 minutes or until the mixture is thickened. Remove from the heat and stir in the molasses, pancake syrup, acesulfame-K, margarine, vanilla extract, spices, and baking soda.

In a separate bowl, use a wire whisk to beat the egg substitute; pour a little of the hot cornmeal into the egg and beat together. Then pour the beaten egg into the larger pan and whisk together.

Pour the mixture into a ½-gallon (2 L) ovenproof baking dish that has been coated with non-stick cooking spray. Set it in a pan of hot water that comes halfway up the side of the dish. Pour the remaining ½ C (125 mL) of milk over the top, but do not stir it in. Bake in a preheated 275°F (140°C) oven for approximately 2½ hours.

Yield: 10 servings **Exchange:** 1 bread
Each serving contains:
Calories: 88 Fiber: trace
Sodium: 95 mg Cholesterol: 1 mg

Scandinavian Pudding

This is a variation of klappgrot, *the traditional Scandinavian dessert.*

6 oz.	frozen apple juice concentrate	180 g
2½ C	water	625 mL
4 T	farina	60 mL
8 oz.	pineapple juice, unsweetened (from a can of crushed pineapple)	240 g

Mix the apple juice and water in a saucepan. Bring to a rapid boil. Stir the mixture while gradually adding the farina. Cook gently for five minutes or so and remove from the heat. Beat by hand or with an electric mixer until the mixture is smooth. Fold in the pineapple. Pour into individual pudding dishes; chill.

Yield: 6 servings **Exchange:** 1 fruit
Each serving contains:
Calories: 88 Fiber: trace
Sodium: 33 mg Cholesterol: 0

Lemon Cake Pudding

This is a tangy, moist cake that you can proudly present at a social event. The beaten egg whites make it rise high.

1 T	margarine or butter, melted	15 mL
2 T	sugar	30 mL
10 pkts	concentrated acesulfame-K	10 pkts
1 t	vanilla extract	5 mL
⅓ C	egg substitute	90 mL
⅓ C	lemon juice	90 mL
2 t	grated lemon peel	10 mL
¼ C	flour	90 mL
1 C	nonfat milk	250 mL
2 drops	yellow food coloring (optional)	2 drops
2	egg whites	2
⅛ t	cream of tartar	.5 mL

Use an electric mixer to beat together the melted margarine, sugar, acesulfame-K, vanilla extract, and egg substitute until smooth. Then add the lemon juice, lemon peel, flour, milk, and food coloring, if desired. Be sure it's well blended.

In a separate bowl, using clean, dry beaters, beat the egg whites until stiff. Add the cream of tartar and beat until stiff. Add a small amount to the lemon batter to lighten it. Then use a rubber spatula to gently fold the remaining egg whites into the batter. Pour it into an ovenproof baking dish that has been coated with non-stick cooking spray. Put this dish into a larger oven pan that has hot water in it. Put it into a preheated 350°F (180°C) oven for 40 minutes. Serve hot or cold

Yield: 8 servings   **Exchange:** ½ milk
Each serving contains:
Calories: 59   Fiber: trace
Sodium: 50 mg   Cholesterol: trace

Cherry-Covered Chocolate

So easy, yet it tastes wonderful. Great for people with a sweet tooth.

1 box	sugar-free instant chocolate pudding	1 box
1¾ C	nonfat milk	440 mL
1 pkg (4 oz.)	sugar-free cherry gelatin	1 pkg (125g)
½ C	boiling water	125 mL
4 oz.	nonfat, no sugar vanilla yogurt	125 g

1 (16 oz.) can	cherries with no sugar or syrup, well drained	1 (450 g) can
2 t	concentrated aspartame	10 mL
½ t	vanilla extract	2.5 mL

Use an electric mixer to combine the chocolate pudding and nonfat milk. Mix until thickened. Spoon into six fancy glasses, such as wine goblets. Set aside. Dissolve the cherry gelatin in the boiling water and stir well. Put the yogurt, drained cherries, aspartame, vanilla extract, and dissolved gelatin into a food processor or blender. Combine for a few seconds or until smooth. Pour the cherry mixture carefully over the chocolate pudding and chill until set.

Yield: 6 servings   **Exchange:** 1 bread + ½ fruit
Each serving contains:
Calories: 105   Fiber: 0
Sodium: 280 mg   Cholesterol: 1.5 mg

Hawaiian Custard

This is one of Karin's grandmother's recipes updated with acesulfame-K. It's wonderfully sweet and creamy.

2 C	skim milk	500 mL
6 pkts	concentrated acesulfame-K	6 pkts
⅓ C	tapioca	90 mL
¼ C	egg substitute	60 mL
1 T	cold water	15 mL
1 C	drained, unsweetened crushed pineapple	250 g

Heat the milk over boiling water in the top of a double boiler. Add the acesulfame-K and tapioca and bring to a boil, stirring occasionally. (If you do not have a double boiler, stir constantly to avoid burning the milk.) With an electric mixer, beat the egg substitute, add cold water, and beat again. Pour the hot mixture over the egg mixture, then return it to the top of a double boiler and cook a moment, stirring constantly. When smooth and thick, beat in the crushed pineapple. Chill thoroughly and serve in dessert cups.

Yield: 8 servings   **Exchange:** 1 fruit
Each serving contains:
Calories: 62   Fiber: trace
Sodium: 50 mg   Cholesterol: 1 mg

Prune-Rice Pudding

This dessert takes a while to make, so get it started when you're in the kitchen anyway. It's actually very little work and well worth the time.

2½ C	pitted prunes	625 mL
1 C	water	250 mL
⅓ C	uncooked regular white rice	90 mL
2 C	milk, scalded	500 mL
3 pkts	concentrated acesulfame-K	3 pkts
1 t	vanilla extract	5 mL
3	egg yolks, slightly beaten	3
2 t	cinnamon	10 mL
3	egg whites	3

In a saucepan cook the prunes and water for 25 minutes. Meanwhile cook the rice, milk, and acesulfame-K for about an hour over boiling water in a covered double boiler. Remove from the heat; stir in the vanilla and egg yolks. Arrange the prunes with ⅓ C (90 mL) of their liquid over the bottom of a 1½ quart (1.5 L) shallow baking dish and sprinkle with the cinnamon. Beat the egg whites until stiff but not dry; partially fold into the rice mixture, leaving some egg white fluffs still intact. Spoon the mixture over the prunes. Bake for 30 minutes in a 350°F (180°C) oven. Serve warm.

Yield: 8 servings   **Exchange:** 2 breads
Each serving contains:
Calories: 165   Fiber: 4 g
Sodium: 58 mg   Cholesterol: 104 mg

Thanksgiving Pudding

This pudding is so low in calories and fat, it's easy to fit in with any meal.

1 (15 oz.)	can pumpkin	1 (425 g) can
2 t	pumpkin pie spice	10 mL
2 t	olive oil	10 mL
1 T	fructose	15 mL
2 t	vanilla extract	10 mL
7 pkts	concentrated acesulfame-K	7 pkts
1 C	skim milk	250 mL
4	egg whites	4

Put the pumpkin, pumpkin pie spice, olive oil, fructose, vanilla extract, and acesulfame-K into a mixing bowl; use a wire whisk to mix completely.

In a small saucepan heat the milk just to the boiling point. Whisk into the pumpkin mixture. In a separate small bowl use an electric mixer to heat the egg whites. Fold the egg whites into the pumpkin-milk mixture. Be sure it is well mixed.

Pour the mixture into 10 separate custard cups that have been coated with non-stick cooking spray. Place the filled custard cups into one very large or two medium ovenproof pans. Carefully pour boiling water into the baking pan(s), taking care that water doesn't spill into the filled cups.

Bake in a preheated 375°F (190°C) oven for 35 minutes. A knife inserted in the center of each custard should come out clean. Chill before serving.

Yield: 10 servings   **Exchange:** ½ bread
Each serving contains:
Calories: 43   Fiber: 2 g
Sodium: 35 mg   Cholesterol: trace

Vanilla Pudding

Our friend Joan wondered why this pudding didn't taste like the instant, store-bought kind until she realized that the sweet taste was the same, but this one happily lacked the salty flavor the high sodium content gave the supermarket product.

2 C	skim milk	500 mL
2 T	margarine or butter	30 mL
3 T	cornstarch	45 mL
2 T	sugar	30 mL
3 pkts	concentrated acesulfame-K	3 pkts
1	egg, or equivalent egg substitute	1
1 T	vanilla extract	15 mL

Heat the milk and margarine over simmering water in the top of a double boiler. In a bowl, mix together the cornstarch, sugar, and acesulfame-K. Add the egg or egg substitute and blend well. Add the vanilla and blend. Pour the cornstarch mixture into the warm milk. Mix with a wire whisk over simmering water until the mixture is thick. A good way to know if it's done is to look for wire whisk patterns; if they stay in the pudding, it's done. Cool the pudding before serving.

Yield: 4 servings   **Exchange:** 1 milk + 1 fat
Each serving contains:
Calories: 147   Fiber: trace
Sodium: 79 mg   Cholesterol: 2 mg

Tapioca Pudding

Very creamy and satisfying.

3 C	skim milk	750 mL
¼ C	quick-cooking (instant) tapioca	125 mL
¼ t	salt (optional)	1 mL
¼ C	egg substitute	60 mL
1	egg white, beaten	1
1 t	vanilla extract	5 mL
2½ t	concentrated aspartame	7 mL

Whisk together the milk, tapioca, salt (optional), egg substitute, and beaten egg white in the top of a double boiler. Heat the water in the lower part to boiling. Cover the top part and cook for five minutes while stirring. Remove from the heat; add the vanilla extract and aspartame. The pudding will thicken as it cools.

Yield: 6 servings   **Exchange:** 1 bread
Each serving contains:
Calories: 79   Fiber: 0
Sodium: 93 mg   Cholesterol: 2 mg

Creamed Apple Tapioca

Luscious and sweet, this is a very satisfying dessert.

2 T	tapioca	30 mL
3 C	skim milk	750 mL
½ C	egg substitute	125 mL
6 pkts	concentrated acesulfame-K	6 pkts
6	apples	6
1 t	nutmeg	5 mL
1 t	cinnamon	5 mL

Cook the tapioca in the milk until it reaches a full boil. Then add the beaten egg substitute and acesulfame-K; stir and remove at once from the heat. Peel and quarter the apples, put them in a casserole dish, and sprinkle them with spices, stirring to coat evenly. Pour the tapioca mixture over them and bake at 325°F (160°C) for 45 minutes or until the apples are soft.

Yield: 6 servings   **Exchange:** 2 breads
Each serving contains:
Calories: 147   Fiber: 4 g
Sodium: 106 mg   Cholesterol: 2 mg

Chocolate Pudding

This recipe is so easy. You are sure to prefer it to boxed pudding. It's much lower in sodium too.

¼ C	sugar	60 mL
3 pkts	concentrated acesulfame-K	3 pkts
2 T	unsweetened cocoa powder	30 mL
3 T	cornstarch	45 mL
2 C	nonfat milk	500 mL
1 t	vanilla extract	5 mL

Combine the sugar, acesulfame-K, cocoa, and cornstarch in a saucepan. Add about ½ C (125 mL) milk. Stir with a wire whisk until dissolved and the mixture is smooth. Add the remaining milk and vanilla extract. Cook, stirring occasionally until thick, about 5 minutes. Cool before serving.

Yield: 4 servings   **Exchange:** 1 bread + ½ fruit
Each serving contains:
Calories: 118   Fiber: trace
Sodium: 81 mg   Cholesterol: 2 mg

Creamy Pudding

Our diabetic friends were really impressed with this pudding, especially those who are the most careful about restricting calories and fat.

1 (8 oz.)can	crushed pineapple, unsweetened	1 (240 mL) can
1 pkg.	unflavored gelatin	1 pkg.
¼ C	water	60 mL
1 T	concentrated aspartame	15 mL
1 t	vanilla extract	5 mL
1 C	nonfat milk	250 mL

Drain the liquid from the canned pineapple into a saucepan; sprinkle the gelatin over it to soften. Bring to a boil and stir until dissolved. Use a blender or food processor to combine with all the other ingredients. Pour into individual dishes. Chill until set.

Yield: 8 servings   **Exchange:** ½ milk
Each serving contains:
Calories: 31   Fiber: trace
Sodium: 17 mg   Cholesterol: trace

Grapefruit Snow Pudding

This is a tart, light pudding that's perfect after a heavy meal.

1 pkt	unsweetened gelatin	1 pkt
¼ C	cold water	60 mL
¼ C	boiling water	60 mL
¼ C	orange juice	60 mL
1 T	lemon juice	15 mL
¾ C	grapefruit, chopped	190 mL
4 pkts	concentrated acesulfame-K	4 pkts
2	egg whites	2
1	grapefruit, cut into sections (optional)	1

Soak the gelatin in the cold water for about five minutes; add the boiling water, then add the acesulfame-K. Stir to dissolve the gelatin. Add the fruit juices and grapefruit, cut in small pieces. Cool, and when the gelatin begins to stiffen, beat until frothy. In another bowl, beat the egg whites until stiff. Fold them into the grapefruit mixture. Turn into a bowl and chill. When serving, garnish with sections of grapefruit.

Yield: 6 servings **Exchange:** free
Each serving contains:
Calories: 27
Sodium: 18 mg
Fiber: trace
Cholesterol: 0

Lemon Pudding

Sometimes your main meal has used up your quota of calories and exchanges. A very light dessert such as this can satisfy the emotional need to have some sweet ending to a meal.

1 env.	unflavored gelatin, unsweetened	1 env.
2 T	cold water	30 mL
½ C	boiling water	125 mL
1½ C	nonfat buttermilk	375 mL
2 t	lemon rind	10 mL
2 t	lemon juice	10 mL
2 t	concentrated aspartame	10 mL
2 drops	yellow food coloring (optional)	2 drops

In a large mixing bowl, sprinkle the gelatin over the cold water to soften. Let sit for a few minutes. Pour boiling water over it and stir until completely dissolved. Add the remaining ingredients and whisk together. Pour into five individual pudding dishes that have been sprayed very lightly with non-stick cooking spray. The pudding may be served in the individual dishes or unmoulded onto separate plates. This can be served plain or dressed up with a little fresh cut-up fruit. If you keep plain frozen strawberries in your freezer, you can take out one to garnish each serving.

Yield: 5 servings   **Exchange:** ½ milk
Each serving contains:
Calories: 31   Fiber: 0
Sodium: 39 mg   Cholesterol: 1.2 mg

Caramel Pudding

This pudding can be unfolded onto separate little dishes for a fancier look. If you wish, spread a thin layer of fruit puree over the top of the pudding, or do what they do in restaurants: Spread the puree directly onto the serving plate and unfold the moulded pudding on it.

1 env.	unflavored gelatin	1 env.
2 T	cold water	30 mL
¼ C	boiling water with 1 t (5 mL) coffee granules dissolved in it	60 mL
1 t	vanilla extract	5 mL
1½ C	skim milk	375 mL
8 oz.	fat-free, sugar-free, light "Crème Caramel"- flavored yogurt	250 g
1 t	aspartame	5 mL

Sprinkle the gelatin over the cold water; allow it to soften. Add the coffee dissolved in the boiling water and whisk well until the gelatin is completely dissolved. Put the remaining ingredients into a food processor. Blend until smooth. Add the coffee and gelatin mixture and mix well. Pour into individual custard cups that have been coated with non-stick cooking spray. Chill until set.

Yield: 8 servings   **Exchange:** ½ milk
Each serving contains:
Calories: 32   Fiber: 0
Sodium: 43 mg   Cholesterol: 1.3 mg

Pineapple Mousse

Karin's mother served this at a dinner party that included diabetic and non-diabetic friends. It was a great success, and it's so quick to make.

1 (20 oz.) can	pineapple, packed in juice, drained	1 (625 mL) can
2 T	fructose	30 mL
1 C	evaporated skim milk, chilled	250 mL
1 env.	unflavored gelatin	1 env.
1 T	lemon juice	15 mL

Puree the pineapple in a blender or food processor. Add the fructose; stir. Set aside. In a mixing bowl, whip the evaporated milk until thick and creamy. In the top of a double boiler, sprinkle the gelatin over the lemon juice. Let stand 3–5 minutes. Stir over hot water until dissolved. Stir the gelatin into the whipped milk. Fold the pineapple mixture into the milk. Spoon into dessert dishes. Chill until set.

Yield: 16 servings   **Exchange:** 1 milk
Each serving contains:
Calories: 51   Fiber: trace
Sodium: 85 mg   Cholesterol: 0

Yogurt Moulds

Make one of the fruit toppings from this book to pour over your yogurt. Add a dollop of your favorite whipped topping.

2 env.	flavored gelatin	2 env.
3 T	water	45 mL
2 C	nonfat plain yogurt, chilled	500 mL
2 t	strawberry extract	10 mL
1 t	almond extract	5 mL

In the top of a double boiler, sprinkle the gelatin over the water and let it stand for 1–5 minutes, until softened. Stir until dissolved. Heat over boiling water. Whisk into the yogurt. Add strawberry and almond extracts. Mix well. Then pour into individual dessert dishes. Chill until set.

Yield: 4 servings   **Exchange:** 1 milk
Each serving contains:
Calories: 64   Fiber: 0
Sodium: 76 mg   Cholesterol: 0

Black Cherry Gelatin

A much more subtle flavor than boxed gelatin from the supermarket, this can use any flavor of sugar-free soda, including ginger ale.

1 env.	flavored gelatin	1 env.
¼ C	cold water	60 mL
2 pkts	concentrated acesulfame-K	2 pkts
2 C	sugar-free black cherry soda	500 mL

Sprinkle the gelatin over the water in the top of a double boiler. Let stand for 5 minutes. Meanwhile, in another bowl, combine the remaining ingredients. Stir the gelatin over hot water until dissolved. Pour into the black cherry mixture. Chill until set. Garnish with fresh fruit slices if desired.

Yield: 4 servings   **Exchange:** free
Each serving contains:
Calories: 7 servings   Fiber: trace
Sodium: 22 mg   Cholesterol: 0

Fast Mocha Aspic

The name says it all. This easy-to-make recipe is light and delightful after a summer meal.

½ C	nonfat milk	125 mL
1 env. (1 T)	unflavored gelatin	1 env. (15 mL)
½ C	cold coffee	125 mL
3 T	sugar	45 mL
3 T	unsweetened cocoa powder (such as Hershey's)	45 mL
1 t	vanilla extract	5 mL
1 t	crushed ice	5 mL

Pour the milk into a small saucepan and heat it gently until very hot but not boiling. Combine the milk and gelatin in a blender container; blend on high speed for about 30 seconds. Add the coffee, sugar, cocoa, and vanilla; blend for another 30 seconds. Lower the speed and begin adding ice a little at a time (that should take another 30 seconds). Blend on high speed for 15 seconds. Chill in individual dishes for at least 30 minutes before serving.

Yield: 4 servings   **Exchange:** 1 bread
Each serving contains:
Calories: 79   Fiber: 0
Sodium: 41 mg   Cholesterol: trace

Swedish Citrus Fromage

This is so fast and easy to "whip" up, and your friends and family will love it. It's especially good after spaghetti and meatballs.

2 t	unflavored, unsweetened gelatin	10 mL
2 T	water	30 mL
2 T	freshly squeezed orange juice	30 mL
1 T	fresh lemon juice	15 mL
1 t	grated orange rind	5 mL
4	eggs, separated	4
2 T	sugar (optional)	30 mL
3 pkts	concentrated acesulfame-K	3 pkts

In a small saucepan, combine the gelatin and water. Let stand for five minutes, then cook over low heat, stirring until the gelatin dissolves. Set aside to cool. Mix in the orange juice, lemon juice, and orange rind. Beat the egg yolks and sugar together until thick and light. Add the gelatin mixture and the acesulfame-K and beat. In a separate bowl, beat the egg whites until stiff. Use a rubber spatula to fold gently into the other gelatin mixture. The mixture will be evenly yellow when it is well combined. Spoon into six dessert dishes.

Yield: 6 servings   **Exchange:** 1 fat
Each serving contains:
Calories: 58   Fiber: trace
Sodium: 47 mg   Cholesterol: 183 mg

CHAPTER EIGHT

Frozen Desserts and Toppings

Ice cream! So creamy and sweet and delicious and so convenient. It's too bad it's so full of calories, fat, and sugar that it's pretty much off limits for diabetic meal plans.

Grocery store freezer cases are now loaded with a new generation of ice cream substitutes. Let's take a look at them and their nutritional information. Frozen yogurt comes with and without fat, with and without sugar. Unfortunately, few products are free of both fat and sugar. But you can find some fat-free, sugar-free frozen yogurts if you check out the freezer sections of enough large grocery stores. Are these products close to ice cream? Not really. But they're OK. You'll probably want to add a little something to boost the flavor appeal. By the way, after yogurt is frozen, any living yogurt or acidophilus culture loses its beneficial effect. And some of our diabetic friends tell us that their blood sugar is not adversely affected by eating a very small serving of the frozen yogurts that have no fat but a little sugar.

In addition to the new frozen yogurts, there are many new "ice creams" without sugar; they are sweetened with aspartame. Most of our taste testers liked them. But these products do contain fat; be sure to read the label. So these no-sugar, lower-fat ice creams are not ideal for daily eating.

In this chapter we offer a number of recipes for frozen desserts that can be considered ice cream substitutes. Our frozen desserts share one problem with all other frozen fruit–based recipes: Once such foods are frozen, they form solid lumps from which it is almost impossible to extract one serving. So here is a method we recommend very highly: After you make up any frozen dessert recipe, freeze it in small amounts. (Save and reuse your small yogurt containers for this purpose; ask your friends to save theirs for you.)

Pour your about-to-be-frozen desserts into these small containers, almost but not quite to the top; liquids expand as they freeze, so leave a little room. Shortly before serving, remove one of these little frozen-solid desserts from the freezer. Microwave it for 30 seconds—just long enough to soften it around the edges. Put it into a dish and slice it in half with a table knife. Put each half into a separate dish; stir briefly with a fork. You now have two 4-ounce (125 g) servings. (If you are serving only one person, put half back into the container and return to the freezer.)

We offer a few topping recipes that are good over a frozen dessert or over a plain pudding or angel cake. We recommend highly our Lemon Curd (page 139) and our Lemon Sauce (page 137)!

Banana Sherbet

This frozen dessert is ideal for everyday eating. It's low in calories and exchanges. Enjoy it frequently.

1 C	nonfat, sugar-free banana-cream-pie-flavored yogurt	250 mL
1 C	mashed bananas	250 mL
1 t	concentrated aspartame	5 mL
1 t	vanilla extract	5 mL
½ t	banana extract	2 mL

Combine all the ingredients in a food processor. Pour into two small yogurt containers; freeze for a few hours or overnight.

Yield: 4 servings   **Exchange:** 1 fruit + ½ milk
Each serving contains:
Calories: 104   Fiber: 2 g
Sodium: 38 mg   Cholesterol: 1 mg

Frosty Frozen Dessert

Any fruit can be used in this recipe. We like nectarines for their gentle, natural sweetness.

1	egg white	1
⅓ C	water	90 mL
⅓ C	nonfat dry milk	90 mL
⅓ C	egg substitute	90 mL
⅓ C	measures-like-sugar aspartame	90 mL
¾ C	fruit puree such as nectarines	180 mL

Use an electric mixer to beat together the first three ingredients until a stiff mixture forms. Set aside. Take a separate mixing bowl and beat together all the other ingredients until smooth. Put the bowl of beaten egg whites back under the beaters, then gently beat the fruit-and-egg-substitute mixture into the beaten egg whites. Pour into small yogurt containers and freeze for several hours or overnight.

Yield: 11 servings, ½ C (125 mL) each   **Exchange:** ½ milk
Each serving contains:
Calories: 36   Fiber: 1 g
Sodium: 36 mg   Cholesterol: trace

Frozen Strawberry Yogurt

This recipe works equally well with any frozen or fresh fruit.

1 (8 oz.) pkg	frozen strawberries, no sugar added	1 (226 g) pkg
1½ t	lemon juice	7 mL
2 t	aspartame	10 mL
1 T	vanilla extract	15 mL
1½ C	nonfat yogurt, no sugar added (plain or vanilla)	375 mL

Put fruit in food processor with flavorings. Puree; add yogurt. Freeze in small yogurt containers for easy serving.

Yield: 6 servings   **Exchange:** 1 milk
Each serving contains:
Calories: 76   Fiber: 1.6 g
Sodium: 74 mg   Cholesterol: 0

Very-Low-Calorie Frozen Yogurt

The type of fruit you pick determines the flavor. Our taste testers preferred blueberries, raspberries, and fresh peaches. Using gelatin and lots of crushed ice makes them very, very low in calories and exchanges.

1 env.	plain gelatin	1 env.
2 T	cold water	30 mL
⅓ C	boiling water	90 mL
1 C	nonfat yogurt no sugar added (any flavor)	250 mL
2 t	aspartame	10 mL
1 t	vanilla or almond extract	5 mL
1 C	fresh or frozen berries or cut-up fruit (with no sugar added)	250 mL
2½ C	crushed ice	625 mL

Sprinkle the gelatin over the cold water; let it sit for a few minutes to soften. Pour in the boiling water and stir until the gelatin is completely dissolved. Combine the yogurt, gelatin, aspartame, extracts, and fruit in a food processor or blender. Mix until well combined. Refrigerate. Just before serving, combine the crushed ice and the chilled mixture in a food processor or blender. Blend together until creamy.

Yield: 10 servings   **Exchange:** free
Each serving contains:
Calories: 21   Fiber: trace
Sodium: 16 mg   Cholesterol: 0

Couldn't-Be-Easier Frozen Yogurt

This recipe is almost not a recipe. Just place a container of yogurt in the freezer and leave until frozen. Coffee-flavored yogurt is wonderful frozen. Carefully read labels at the grocery store; be sure to buy nonfat yogurt sweetened only with aspartame. Coffee frozen yogurt is even better with a tablespoon of dietetic pancake syrup.

Yield: 2 servings   **Exchange:** ½ milk
Each serving contains:
Calories: 53   Fiber: 0
Sodium: 73 mg   Cholesterol: 0

Almost Ice Cream

Using cottage cheese and dry milk powder together adds a creamy texture to this. It is very important to process the cottage cheese for the full two minutes. If you cheat on the time, cottage cheese curds may spoil the effect.

1 env.	plain gelatin	1 env.
2 T	cold water	30 mL
1 C	boiling water	250 mL
1⅓ C	cottage cheese	340 mL
3 T	nonfat dry milk	45 mL
1 T	concentrated aspartame	15 mL
2 t	vanilla extract	10 mL
2 t	lemon juice	10 mL
⅓ C	ice water	90 mL
1 C	fruit (fresh or frozen without sugar)	250 mL

Sprinkle the gelatin on the cold water; set aside for a few minutes. Pour boiling water over the gelatin and stir until completely dissolved. Put the gelatin, cottage cheese, dry milk, aspartame, vanilla extract, and lemon juice into a food processor. Process for a full two minutes. Then put the mixture into a bowl and chill until the gelatin has set. Keep it refrigerated until shortly before serving time. Then put it into a food processor or blender with the ice water and fruit. Process for a few seconds until blended but not frothy. Serve immediately.

Yield: 8 servings per 4 C (1 L)   **Exchange:** ½ milk
Each serving contains:
Calories: 53   Fiber: trace
Sodium: 17 mg   Cholesterol: 4 mg

Pear Ice Not-Cream

This frosty pear treat is another dessert low enough in calories to enjoy often.

4 C	pear slices (about 3 large or 4 medium pears)	1 L
2½ C	water	625 mL
3 pkts	acesulfame-K	3 pkts
1 t	concentrated clear vanilla extract	5 mL
½ t	imitation brandy flavor	2 mL
1 T	aspartame	15 mL

Combine the pear slices, water, acesulfame-K, and extracts in a saucepan over medium heat. When it first comes to a boil, reduce the heat and simmer for half an hour. Turn off the heat. Stir in the aspartame. Pour into a food processor or blender and puree. Then pour into small containers and freeze until solid. Just before serving, allow to defrost slightly.

Yield: 8 servings   **Exchange:** 1 fruit
Each serving contains:
Calories: 49   Fiber: 2 g
Sodium: 0   Cholesterol: 0

Icy Grapes

What could be easier? People who try these are amazed.

Wash the grapes and place them in the freezer for several hours or overnight. Serve in fancy wine glasses.

Yield: **Exchange:** 1 fruit
½ C (125 mL) grapes contains:
Calories: 54   Fiber: trace
Sodium: 3 mg   Cholesterol: 0

CHAPTER NINE

Desserts for Special Occasions

In this chapter we present desserts that take a little more effort but that are spectacular. None requires special skill, however. In the case of soufflés, the only tricky part is that they need to be served shortly after they come out of the oven. The trifle recipe makes more than a small family would eat at one time.

Many people enjoy serving special desserts at parties or when the whole family gathers together. With some of the recipes in this chapter, we suggest you get people to join in on the fun of assembling. For example, you might have an evening get-together where people assemble their own napoleons.

Grand Marnier Soufflé for Six

The tricky part of soufflés is to serve them right away when they are all puffed up.

2 T	margarine or butter	30 mL
2½ T	regular all-purpose flour	37 mL
¾ C	skim milk	190 Ml
1 pkt	concentrated acesulfame-K	1 pkt
2	egg yolks, beaten	2
3	egg whites	3
⅛ t	cream of tartar	.5 mL
3 T	Grand Marnier	45 mL

In a saucepan melt the margarine or butter and remove it from the heat. Stir in the flour and milk; cook, stirring over medium heat, until thickened and smooth. Stir in the acesulfame-K; cool slightly; add egg yolks.

In a medium bowl, beat the egg whites until foamy; add the cream of tartar, beating until stiff peaks form when the beater is raised. Gently fold the egg yolk mixture and Grand Marnier into the egg whites. Turn into a one-quart soufflé dish or casserole coated with non-stick cooking spray.

Bake for 10 minutes in a preheated 450°F (230°C) oven, then turn down the heat to 325°F (160°C) and bake 15 minutes longer. Serve immediately.

Yield: 6 servings   **Exchange:** 1 fat + 1 bread
Each serving contains:
Calories: 122   Fiber: trace
Sodium: 27 mg   Cholesterol: 34 mg

Grand Marnier Soufflé for Eight

Grand Marnier is a special liqueur. Those who prefer to avoid alcohol, even when it cooks out, can make this soufflé without it. Those who want to try the Grand Marnier may want to buy a very small ("nip") bottle, as the liqueur is expensive.

1½ C	nonfat milk	375 mL
2 T	margarine or butter	30 mL
3 T	flour	45 mL
¼ C	egg substitute	60 mL
2 T	fructose	30 mL
⅓ C	measures-like-sugar saccharin	90 mL
7 pkts	acesulfame-K	7 pkts
2 t	vanilla extract	10 mL
1½ t	orange extract	7 mL
3 T	orange-flavored liqueur such as Grand Marnier (optional)	45 mL
4	egg whites	4
½ t	cream of tartar	2 mL
2 T	measures-like-sugar aspartame	30 mL

Heat the milk just to the boiling point and set it aside. In a separate saucepan, melt the margarine over low heat and add flour. Stir together for two minutes over low-to-medium heat, stirring constantly. Turn off the heat. Whisk in the hot milk, stirring constantly. Cook over medium heat, until the mixture thickens. Turn off the heat. Slowly stir in the egg substitute. Then stir in the fructose, saccharin, acesulfame-K, vanilla and orange extracts, and liqueur, if using. Set aside.

In a separate bowl, beat the egg whites and cream of tartar and continue beating until stiff. Mix a small amount of the beaten egg whites into the milk mixture to lighten it. Then use a rubber spatula to fold in the rest of the beaten egg whites. Pour the mixture into a soufflé dish that has been coated with non-stick cooking spray. Bake in a preheated 375°F (190°C) oven for 20 minutes. Do not overbake. As soon as the soufflé is out of the oven, use a small sieve to dust aspartame over the top.

Yield: 8 servings   **Exchange:** ½ fruit + ½ meat
Each serving contains:
Calories: 78   Fiber: trace
Sodium: 97 mg   Cholesterol: trace

Hot Apple Soufflé

This makes the house smell wonderful when it's baking and tastes great, too.

½ C	margarine or butter	125 mL
½ C	flour	125 mL
2 C	cold skim milk	500 mL
2 T	granulated sugar	30 mL
1 pkt	concentrated acesulfame-K	1 pkt
	grated peel from ½ lemon	
2	medium apples	2
4	eggs, separated	4
2 T	slivered toasted almonds	30 mL

About 2¼ hours before serving, melt the margarine in a medium saucepan; stir in the flour, then the milk. Cook, stirring constantly, until smooth and thickened. Blend in the sugar, acesulfame-K, and lemon peel; let cool slightly, stirring occasionally.

Meanwhile, wash, pare, and core the apples, then cut each into about 10 lengthwise wedges. Arrange them evenly over the bottom of a casserole which measures 8 C (2 L) to the brim. Beat the egg whites until stiff. Blend the yolks into the flour-milk mixture, then carefully fold in the egg whites. Pour this mixture over the apples, then sprinkle it with almonds. Bake in a preheated 325°F (160°C) oven for 1¼ hours or until light brown and firm. Serve at once.

> **Yield:** 8 servings.   **Exchange:** 1 bread + ½ meat + 1 fat
> **Each serving contains:**
> Calories: 229   Fiber: 1 g
> Sodium: 67 mg   Cholesterol: 138 mg

Chocolate Soufflé

This is absolutely wonderful.

½ C	unsweetened cocoa powder	125 mL
2 T	powdered sugar	30 mL
½ C	measures-like-sugar saccharin	125 mL
7 pkts	concentrated acesulfame-K	7 pkts
2 T	cornstarch	30 mL
dash	salt (optional)	dash
½ C	nonfat milk	125 mL
½ C	water	125 mL
4	egg whites	4
½ t	cream of tartar	2 mL

¼ C	egg substitute	60 mL
1 t	vanilla extract	5 mL
2 T	measures-like-sugar aspartame	30 mL

Sift the cocoa, sugar, saccharin and acesulfame-K, salt, and cornstarch together twice. Put them in the top of a double boiler and add the nonfat milk and water. Whisk constantly while cooking until the mixture is smooth and thick, about eight minutes. Remove from the heat. Beat the egg whites with an electric mixer until they hold their shape; add the cream of tartar, and continue beating until stiff peaks form. Pour the egg substitute and vanilla extract into the chocolate mixture. Mix. Add a small amount of the beaten egg whites into the chocolate mixture to lighten. Then use a rubber spatula to fold in the rest of the egg whites.

Pour into a 6 C (1.5 L) soufflé dish that has been coated with non-stick cooking spray. Bake in a preheated 400°F (200°C) oven for 20 minutes. Do not overcook; the center will be a little runny to make a sauce. As soon as the soufflé is out of the oven, dust aspartame over the top.

Yield: 8 servings   **Exchange:** ½ bread
Each serving contains:
Calories: 54   Fiber: 0
Sodium: 84 mg   Cholesterol: trace

Berry Soufflé

A lovely and impressive soufflé that tastes as good as it looks.

1¾ C	mixed red berries (fresh or unsweetened frozen, thawed and drained)	440 mL
1 T	Chambord or fruit-flavored liqueur (optional) or 2 t (10 mL) strawberry extract	15 mL
5	egg whites	5

In a blender or food processor, puree the berries and liqueur. In a mixing bowl, beat the egg whites until stiff but not dry. Fold the puree into the egg whites. Spoon the mixture into a two-quart soufflé dish coated with non-stick cooking spray. Place the soufflé dish on a cooking sheet and bake for 35–30 minutes at 350°F (180°C). Serve immediately.

Yield: 6 servings   **Exchange:** ½ milk
Each serving contains:
Calories: 31   Fiber: 2 g
Sodium: 42 mg   Cholesterol: 0

Oat Bran Pancakes for Oat Bran Cake

These pancakes can be served as part of a special brunch, or, of course, at any meal. Please try them also for the Oat Bran Cake, on page 17.

1 C	oat bran hot cereal, uncooked	250 mL
½ C	whole-wheat flour	125 mL
2 pkts	concentrated acesulfame-K	2 pkts
2 t	baking powder	10 mL
1 C	nonfat milk	250 mL
1 T	vegetable oil	15 mL
2	egg whites, slightly beaten	2

Combine the oat bran, flour, acesulfame-K, and baking powder. In another bowl, combine the remaining ingredients. Pour the wet mixture into the dry and mix until moistened. Pour ½ C (125 mL) batter for each pancake onto a medium-high griddle coated with non-stick cooking spray. Turn when bubbles form on the surface. Serve with fruit topping.

Yield: 4 servings   **Exchange:** 2 breads + ½ fat
Each serving contains:
Calories: 213   Fiber: 9 g
Sodium: 255 mg   Cholesterol: 1 mg

Unbelievable Napoleons

Did you ever think you could make napoleons as wonderful as the ones in the bakery? You can, and they're easy, too.

Napoleon Pastry

| 4 sheets | fillo dough | 4 sheets |

If you are unfamiliar with how to work with fillo dough, first read the general instructions on pages 74–75.

Take one sheet of fillo dough and spread it flat; coat with butter-flavored non-stick vegetable cooking spray. Fold the dough in half and spray it again. Fold it again; the sheet is now one-quarter of its original size. Using scissors, cut it into four pieces. You now have four small pieces, each of which is four layers thick. Carefully lift each onto a cookie sheet that has been sprayed with non-stick vegetable cooking spray. Make as many sections as you need. Plan to stack the dough four pieces high for a super napoleon; in this case, one sheet of fillo makes one napoleon, with fillings. Bake in a preheated 375°F (190°C) oven for approximately six minutes. The dough should be lightly browned but not burnt. Use a pancake turner to lift each piece off, and place each on a wire rack to cool. Store in an airtight container. The analysis is for a four-layer napoleon, unfilled. Be sure to add the extra calories and exchanges for the fillings.

Yield: 4 napoleons   **Exchange:** 2 breads
Each napoleon contains:
Calories: 180   Fiber: 1 g
Sodium: 120 mg   Cholesterol: 0

Chocolate Napoleon Filling

This filling is great for cream puffs, too.

| ½ C | nonfat milk | 125 mL |
| 1 pkg | chocolate sugar-free instant pudding | 1 pkg |

Pour the milk into a bowl. Add the pudding mix and mix well. Using an electric mixer is an easy way to do this. Spread 2 T (30 mL) as a chocolate layer.

Yield: 12 servings   **Exchange:** free
2 T (30 mL) contains:
Calories: 21   Fiber: 0
Sodium: 1226 mg   Cholesterol: trace

Napoleon Fillings

Having a napoleon party for a special occasion is great fun. Let people assemble their own by setting out a choice of fillings and shells. Lemon curd is good, as is pudding. For a very quick filling, use instant, sugar-free pudding mix, but use 1⅓ C (340 mL) of skim milk instead of the full amount called for. Whipped cream substitutes are also nice. Slices of strawberries, kiwis, or bananas add a festive touch. To keep cut fruit looking fresh, sprinkle a little lemon juice on it. Add a sprinkle of aspartame if you like. A few frozen blueberries add color and flavor.

Trifle

Trifle is among the easiest desserts to make, and it really gets compliments. Gather your ingredients and assemble them in a showy bowl, sit back, and wait for the oohs and aahs. We've given you two trifle recipes: one for traditional fruit trifle and one for a chocolate trifle that is wonderful. As with all our recipes, everyone will be happy with these desserts, not just diabetics.

Fruit Trifle

Trifles are usually served in large, straight-sided, clear-glass pedestal bowls. A traditional trifle consists of layers of brandy-soaked cake, fruit, pudding, and whipped cream. Trifles look beautiful and are delicious. When you're serving a crowd, a trifle is sure to please.

To assemble a trifle, use angel food cake, hot-milk sponge cake, or yellow cake. Recipes for these cakes are in Chapter Two. Tear the cake into 2 × 2-inch (5 × 5 cm) bits and spread some on the bottom of the trifle bowl. Drop on a layer of sugar-free vanilla pudding, then add a layer of fruit. Blueberries, kiwis, and strawberries make an attractive and delicious combination. Then add a layer of sugar-free whipped topping. After the topping layer, start again with cake. Make as many layers as you have ingredients and room in the dish. Or, make individual trifles with pudding, fruit, topping, and a bit of leftover cake. Assemble the layers in wine or champagne glasses for a festive look.

Here are a few tips to make trifles suitable for people on diabetic diets:

*Most "low-sugar/ low-fat" whipped toppings dissolve after half an hour or so. That means you need to assemble the trifle close to serving time.

*Use only ingredients that you know are suitable. Stay away from frozen or canned puddings or fruit with sugar.

*Bananas need to be tossed in lemon juice if you're using banana slices. Otherwise, they turn dark, gooey, and unappetizing.

*Traditional trifle recipes call for cake soaked in brandy or other liqueur. We leave that out and instead add brandy extract to the pudding.

Chocolate Trifle

This is a chocoholic's dream. A chocolate trifle is nontraditional but a great favorite nonetheless. To make a chocolate trifle, use the same clear, straight-sided, glass pedestal bowl and assemble in layers, but use chocolate cake, chocolate pudding, bittersweet sauce, and whipped topping.

Try the Devil's Food Cake, on page 22. It's an excellent choice for the cake layers. Any sugar-free whipped topping is fine: Low-fat topping is good, but remember that most dissolve in a short time, so assemble the trifle just before serving.

Use the Chocolate Pudding recipe, on page 115, for your pudding layers, or the boxed, sugar-free kind. Then drizzle on one of the chocolate, bittersweet, or sweet sauces from this book, and enjoy.

Mousse au Chocolat

This is a genuinely rich mousse. Very creamy and satisfying. We used a "diabetic" candy bar with sorbitol.

2 t	unflavored gelatin	10 mL
¼ C	cold water	60 mL
⅓ C	unsweetened cocoa powder	90 mL
1 t	cornstarch	5 mL
15 pkts	concentrated acesulfame-K	15 pkts
1 t	vanilla extract	5 mL
¼ C	skim milk	60 mL
1 (2½ oz.)	milk chocolate bar made without chocolate	1 (71 g)
6 T	nonfat cream cheese	90 mL
4	egg whites	4
¼ t	cream of tartar	1 mL

Sprinkle the gelatin over the cold water to soften. In a saucepan, whisk together the cocoa, cornstarch, acesulfame-K, vanilla extract, and milk. Cook over medium heat for a few minutes, stirring with a wire whisk. Remove from the heat. Use a food processor or blender to chop the chocolate bar into small pieces; stir the chocolate into the cocoa mixture until smooth. Stir in the softened gelatin. Heat the cream cheese over low heat or in the microwave oven until softened. Add small amounts of the chocolate mixture to the softened cream cheese. Whisk until it is smooth and creamy and no small lumps remain. Use a rubber spatula to add this cream cheese–chocolate mixture back into the saucepan and whisk well to combine with the remaining chocolate.

Set the saucepan into a large bowl chilled with ice cubes and ice water to cool and thicken. In a separate bowl beat the egg whites until foamy; add the cream of tartar and continue beating until stiff peaks form. Put a small amount of the chocolate mixture into the beaten egg whites to lighten. Then use a rubber spatula to fold the rest of the egg whites into the chocolate mixture. Pour into eight small (½ C or 125 mL) serving dishes and refrigerate until set.

Yield: 8 servings   **Exchange:** ½ milk + ½ fat
Each serving contains:
Calories: 81   Fiber: 0
Sodium: 147 mg   Cholesterol: 3 mg

Cream Puffs

Do you think cream puffs are hard to make? You'll be pleasantly surprised how easy they are. This recipe makes cream puffs as good as the ones in bakeries.

The Puff Pastry

1 C	water	250 mL
⅓ C	canola oil	90 mL
1 C	flour	250 mL
4	eggs or equivalent egg substitute	4
1 t	butter-flavored extract	5 mL
1 t	vanilla extract	5 mL

Heat the water and oil to rolling boil. Lower the heat and add the flour all at once, stirring with a wooden spoon until mixture forms a ball. Remove from the heat. With an electric mixer, beat in the eggs thoroughly, one at a time. Add the butter-flavored extract. Using a spoon, drop 12 cream puffs onto ungreased cookie sheets. Bake in a 400°F (200°C) oven for 10 minutes. Reduce the heat to 350°F (180°C) and bake for 25 minutes longer. Do not remove the cream puffs from the oven until they are quite firm to the touch. Cool the shells away from drafts before filling. To fill, cut horizontally using a sharp knife. If any damp dough remains inside, scoop it out before filling.

Fill the shells with pudding. Top with White Whipped Topping (page 147) and Chocolate Sauce (page 146) or Bittersweet Sauce (page 147).

Yield: 12 cream puffs   **Exchange:** ½ bread + 1 fat
Each cream puff contains:
Calories: 101   Fiber: trace
Sodium: 44 mg   Cholesterol: 0

Crêpes

This recipe makes 14 five-inch (13 cm) crêpes. You can make them in a larger skillet and use strawberry or blueberry topping or a different fruit filling such as fruit-only jam.

1 pkt	concentrated acesulfame-K	1 pkt
1 C	skim milk	250 mL
2 T	safflower oil	30 mL
½ C	egg substitute	125 mL
½ C	flour	125 mL
2 t	baking powder	10 mL
¼ t	vanilla extract	1 mL

Combine all the ingredients in a blender and blend for a minute or so or mix in an electric mixer until the batter is smooth. Heat a small, oiled skillet or crêpe pan until a drop of water "dances" when you splash it on the hot surface. Add ⅓ C (90 mL) of the batter and move the pan around so the batter covers evenly. Cook over medium heat on one side until the edges are browned and there are bubbles throughout the crêpe. Turn and cook on the other side to brown. Spoon one tablespoon (15 mL) of strawberry topping on each crêpe and roll the crêpes up. Top with a dollop of your favorite whipped topping.

Yield: 14 crêpes   **Exchange:** ½ fat
Each crêpe contains:
Calories: 44   Fiber: trace
Sodium: 28 mg   Cholesterol: trace

Crêpes Suzettes Sauce

Crêpes suzettes are wonderful! We offer here a version that is much lower in fat and sweeteners. If you prefer to avoid liqueurs, double the amount of orange extract. You can serve this sauce over your choice of crêpes. Be sure to add together the calories and other values for both the sauce and the crêpe.

¾ C	orange juice	190 mL
1 t	grated orange peel	5 mL
1½ t	cornstarch	7 mL
1 pkt	concentrated acesulfame-K	1 pkt
1 t	margarine or butter	5 mL
1 t	concentrated aspartame	5 mL
½ t	orange extract	2 mL
2 T	orange-flavored liqueur, such as Grand Marnier (optional)	30 mL

In a saucepan whisk together the orange juice, orange peel, cornstarch, and acesulfame-K. Heat to boiling, then immediately reduce the heat and cook over a medium flame, stirring constantly. When the mixture is thickened, turn off the heat.

Stir in the margarine, aspartame, orange extract, and liqueur if desired. Take each crêpe and fold in half, then again, and arrange on a separate plate. Spoon a little crêpes suzettes sauce over each.

Yield: 6 servings   **Exchange:** free
Each serving contains:
Calories: 22   Fiber: trace
Sodium: 7 mg   Cholesterol: 0

No-Fat Crêpes

These crêpes work very well despite the lack of fat. They are easy to cook and easy to roll around fillings. The easiest crêpe fillings are a little nonfat ricotta cheese sweetened with aspartame and nutmeg or flavored applesauce.

1 C	nonfat milk	250 mL
¼ C	egg substitute	60 mL
¾ C	flour	190 mL
2 pkts	acesulfame-K	2 pkts
½ t	cinnamon	2 mL
1 t	sugar	5 mL

Combine all the ingredients in a blender or food processor until smooth. Heat a non-stick omelette pan over medium-high heat. Spoon 2 T (30 mL) batter into the hot pan and roll the pan from side to side to cover the entire surface. When the edges curl away from the sides of the pan, turn the crêpe over. Repeat until all the batter is used. Store crêpes in a covered container with a piece of plastic wrap, waxed paper, or aluminum foil between each crêpe.

Yield: 12 crêpes   **Exchange:** ½ milk
Each crêpe contains:
Calories: 38   Fiber: trace
Sodium: 22 mg   Cholesterol: trace

Traditional Crêpe Filling

Nonfat ricotta cheese makes a nice crêpe filling, especially when flavored with a little nutmeg. Add aspartame if you want it sweeter. Adding a couple of sliced strawberries or raspberries is a nice touch. A whipped topping can also be used.

Raspberry Puree

Raspberry puree is great between layers of napoleons or topping cream puffs or just on nonfat, unsweetened yogurt. You're only limited by your imagination.

1 C   raspberries (fresh or frozen without sugar)   250 mL

Puree the raspberries in a food processor. Spoon into a sieve; with the spoon, push the juice through to remove the seeds. Sweeten to taste with artificial sweetener such as aspartame or acesulfame-K.

> **Yield:** 1 C (250 mL)   **Exchange:** free
> **2 T (30 mL) contain:**
> Calories: 8   Fiber: 0.75 g
> Sodium: 0   Cholesterol: 0

Lemon Sauce

Serve this sauce over ice cream or frozen yogurt or drizzled over angel food cake. It's also great over fruit. It turns an ordinary dessert into an occasion!

⅓ C	fresh lemon juice	90 mL
1 T	grated lemon peel	15 mL
6 pkts	concentrated acesulfame-K	6 pkts
¼ C	egg substitute (or 1 egg)	60 mL
1 T	cornstarch dissolved in	15 mL
	1 T (15 mL) water	
1 t	vanilla extract (clear is nice)	5 mL
1 t	aspartame	5 mL

Combine the lemon juice, lemon peel, and acesulfame-K in a saucepan and simmer. In a separate small bowl use a wire whisk to beat the egg substitute and then blend in the cornstarch-water mixture. Add a little of the hot lemon mixture to the egg and stir to combine. Gradually add the rest of the egg into the saucepan and stir. Cook over medium heat, stirring constantly until thickened. Remove from heat; add the vanilla extract and aspartame. Stir to combine.

> **Yield:** ⅔ C (180 mL) per 11 servings   **Exchange:** free
> **Each serving contains:**
> Calories: 8   Fiber: trace
> Sodium: 7.8 mg   Cholesterol: 0

Magic Touches

In this chapter we offer two types of information. First, we offer a collection of recipes that are themselves ingredients in other recipes. These include prune puree, which you can use to cut way back on fat in baking. Pastry cream and raspberry puree also serve as ingredients in other recipes. Lemon curd and lemon sauce are both great for covering up the taste of artificial sweeteners. But please use fresh lemon juice or you'll lose the magic.

Also in this chapter we offer information about whipped toppings and glazes and other touches that professionals bakers use to make desserts look and taste appealing, and they have all been adapted for diabetic cooking!

Whipped toppings are probably the most commonly served toppings. We offer you several recipes for whipped toppings that are reasonably low in calories and fat. One drawback of prepared packaged mixes and of our own homemade toppings is that they do not have the staying power we have come to expect from whipped toppings. Some of these prepared products come with unhealthy saturated fats such as palm kernel or coconut oil; others are free from such unhealthy "tropical" oils. Some have sugar, while others do not. Read the label before you buy. We would like to add a word here about portion size, using whipped toppings as an example. Cool Whip Lite and similar products are commonly available in the freezer section. On the label we see that a serving is only 20 calories. Great news! But a serving is two tablespoons. Two tablespoons means two level tablespoons. "Two tablespoons" should not give us license to use a large spoon twice to scoop up a generous dollop of whipped topping.

Prune Puree as Fat Replacement

¼ C	unsweetened apple juice	60 mL
1 T	flavoring (vanilla extract or lemon extract or liqueur)	15 mL

Use a food processor to puree all the ingredients. Store the mixture in the refrigerator. Use it as a fat substitute in cooking.

Yield: 1¼ C (310 mL) **Exchange:** free
¼ C (60 mL) contains:
Calories: 13 Fiber: 0.45 g
Sodium: 0.4 mg Cholesterol: 0

Lemon Curd

As good as the expensive version in the fancy container.

⅓ C	fresh lemon juice	90 mL
1 T	cornstarch dissolved in 2 T (30 mL) water	15 mL
7 pkts	concentrated acesulfame-K	7 pkts
¼ C	egg substitute	60 mL
2 t	vanilla extract	10 mL

Put the lemon juice, cornstarch, and acesulfame-K into a small saucepan and whisk together over medium-low heat. Cook gently until the mixture starts to thicken.

In a separate container heat the egg substitute and add it to a small amount of the thickened lemon mixture. Then whisk this mixture into the rest of the lemon mixture in the saucepan. Add the vanilla extract and cook over medium-low heat for one minute.

Yield: 1 C (250 mL)   **Exchange:** free
1 T (15 mL) contains:
Calories: 5   Fiber: trace
Sodium: 9 mg   Cholesterol: 0

Banana Frosting

We used the banana-cream-pie-flavored fat-free, sugar-free yogurt in this recipe, but you can try other flavors as well. Just change the extract to match the yogurt.

4 oz.	nonfat cream cheese	125 mL
4 oz. (½ container)	banana-cream-pie-flavored fat-free, sugar-free yogurt	125 mL
½ t	vanilla extract	2 mL
½ t	banana extract	2 mL
1 T	aspartame	15 mL

Use an electric mixer to combine all ingredients until smooth.

Yield: 16 servings of 1 C (250 mL)   **Exchange:** free
1 T (15 mL) serving contains:
Calories: 9   Fiber: 0
Sodium: 38 mg   Cholesterol: 1 mg

Glaze to Add Sweetness to Cakes and Muffins

This trick comes from aspartame cookbooks.

15 pkts	concentrated aspartame	15 pkts
3 T	boiling water	45 mL
½ t	cinnamon (or your choice of spice)	2 mL

Blend and drizzle over cakes and cookies as they come out of the oven. or brush on with pastry brush to coat more evenly. You may want to use a fork first to poke holes in the pastry to help the glaze penetrate.

Yield: 8 servings   **Exchange:** free
Each serving contains:
Calories: 0   Fiber: 0
Sodium: 0   Cholesterol: 0

Applesauce Frosting

A healthy topping that's also easy to make.

4 oz.	nonfat cream cheese	170 mL
1 t	vanilla extract	5 mL
2 T	unsweetened applesauce	30 mL
1 T	concentrated aspartame	15 mL
1 T	nonfat milk	15 mL

Combine all ingredients and beat with an electric mixer until smooth and creamy.

Yield: 1 C (250 mL)   **Exchange:** free
1 T (15 mL) contains:
Calories: 9   Fiber: trace
Sodium: 36 mg   Cholesterol: 1 mg

Rich Chocolate Frosting

Very satisfying.

½ C	unsweetened cocoa powder	125 mL
⅓ C	measures-like-sugar saccharin	90 mL
½ C	nonfat buttermilk	125 mL
1 t	vanilla extract	5 mL
1 T	measures-like sugar aspartame	15 mL

Combine cocoa and saccharin in a saucepan and whisk in a small amount of buttermilk. Slowly whisk in the remaining buttermilk. Heat over medium heat, whisking constantly. Bring to a boil. Boil for 2 minutes, stirring constantly. When it is thick, remove from heat and stir in vanilla extract and aspartame.

Yield: 1 C (250 mL)   **Exchange:** free
1 T (15 mL) contains:
Calories: 10   Fiber: 0
Sodium: 49 mg   Cholesterol: 0

Chocolate Frosting

The low-fat version is very nice but does not keep as attractively as high-fat frosting.

1 C	nonfat cottage cheese	250 mL
2 T	nonfat cream cheese	30 mL
½ t	vanilla extract	2 mL
½ t	chocolate extract	2 mL
1 T	concentrated aspartame	15 mL
1 T	unsweetened cocoa powder	15 mL

Combine all ingredients in a food processor or blender. Frost just before serving.

Yield: 1 C   **Exchange:** free
1 T (15 mL) contains:
Calories: 14.5   Fiber: 0
Sodium: 223 mg   Cholesterol: 3 mg

Creamy Frosting

A rich, creamy frosting with lemon peel to brighten the flavor.

1 pkg	nonfat cream cheese	1 pkg
¼ C	nonfat yogurt, no sugar added	60 mL
1 T	aspartame	15 mL
1 t	dried lemon peel	5 mL
1 t	vanilla extract	5 mL

Combine all the ingredients and beat with an electric mixer until creamy.

Yield: ¾ C (190 mL)   **Exchange:** free
1 T (15 mL) contains:
Calories: 19   Fiber: 0
Sodium: 93 mg   Cholesterol: 2.7 mg

Creamy Cocoa Frosting

This frosting is great on the Chocolate Tube Cake (page 20) or on the Chocolate Muffins (page 66).

4 oz.	nonfat cream cheese	120 g
3 T	skim milk	45 mL
2 t	concentrated aspartame	10 mL
2 T	unsweetened cocoa powder	30 mL
1 t	cornstarch	5 mL
1 t	vanilla extract	5 mL

Soften the cream cheese in a microwave oven for about 30 seconds. Whisk together the remaining ingredients until smooth. Whisk in the cream cheese.

Yield: 8 servings   **Exchange:** free
Each serving contains:
Calories: 21   Fiber: 0
Sodium: 79 mg   Cholesterol: 2.1 mg

Light Cocoa Frosting

Quick and very satisfying.

1 env.	sugar-free whipped topping mix	1 env.
1 T	unsweetened cocoa powder	15 mL
½ C	ice water	125 mL
1 t	vanilla extract	5 mL

If possible, chill bowl and beaters of an electric mixer. Then combine all ingredients and beat for 4–5 minutes.

Makes enough to frost top and middle of large cake.

Yield: 1 C (250 mL)   **Exchange:** 1 fat
1 T (15 mL) contains:
Calories: 34   Fiber: 0
Sodium: 22 mg   Cholesterol: 0

Toppings

If you'd like to put something on your frozen yogurt or ice cream substitute, ask yourself how many calories and exchanges you can afford to spend. A little Crystal Light adds a festive touch with no calories. Dietetic pancake syrup is another idea. Some are made with saccharin, others are with fructose or sorbitol. Be sure you know how various ingredients affect you before you pour.

Some recipes in this book make good toppings, for example, Lemon Sauce (page 137), Lemon Curd (page 139), and Chocolate Sauce (page 148). Sweetened thickened fruit mixtures can be pie fillings or ice cream toppings. If you are using fruit as a topping, you can use aspartame because the dish will not be heated, as a pie would be. Try unsweetened applesauce with a little aspartame and cinnamon sprinkled on or stirred in.

Wonderful Whipped Cream Substitute

Don't cheat on the time for processing the cottage cheese!

1 C	nonfat cottage cheese	250 mL
1 t	concentrated aspartame	5 mL
½ t	vanilla extract	2 mL

Process the cottage cheese in a food processor for a full 2 minutes. Add aspartame and vanilla extract and process for another minute. Store in the refrigerator up to a few days.

Yield: 1 C (250 mL)   **Exchange:** free
2 T (30 mL) contain:

Calories: 11.5	Fiber: 0
Sodium: 0	Cholesterol: 1 mg

Peach Shortcake Topping

You can serve this over a shortcake-type biscuit, hot milk sponge cake, angel cake, dessert waffles, or crêpes.

4	peaches	4
1½ T	fresh lemon juice	22 mL
1 t	concentrated aspartame	5 mL
¼ t	cinnamon	1 mL

Drop the peaches into boiling water for two minutes to loosen skins. Remove them from hot water; peel, and slice. Place the peaches in a bowl; sprinkle with lemon juice, aspartame, and cinnamon. Stir to combine.

Yield: 6 servings   **Exchange:** free
1 serving contains:

Calories: 25	Fiber: trace
Sodium: trace	Cholesterol: 0

Granola Topping

If you like a crunchy topping on frozen yogurt or other desserts, make up some granola topping and keep it on hand. This is also the recipe we used for our Granola Cheesecake, page 38.

3 C	oatmeal	750 mL
½ C	wheat germ	125 mL
⅔ C	sliced unsalted almonds (optional)	180 mL
1 T	safflower oil	15 mL
2 T	molasses	30 mL
½ C	unsweetened apple juice	125 mL

Mix the oatmeal, wheat germ, and almonds in a lasagna or jelly-roll pan. Heat the remaining ingredients in a saucepan and stir to combine. Drizzle this over the oatmeal mixture, then use a spatula to push the mixture around in the pan until evenly coated. Bake in a 325°F (160°C) oven for about 30 minutes. Then mix again and bake for 10 minutes. The longer you cook it, the crunchier the granola gets. Makes 4½ C (1.125 L).

Yield: 70 T (15 mL) **Exchange:** free
1 T (15 mL) contains:
Calories: 12 Fiber: trace
Sodium: 16 mg Cholesterol: 0

Blueberry Topping

This is a great topping for plain yogurt, ice cream, crêpes, and waffles. You'll be glad to have it on hand. If it seems too thick, heat it a little before serving.

1 (12 oz.)	frozen whole blueberries, no sugar added, thawed	1 (250 mL)pkg
1 T	cornstarch	15 mL
½ C	fruit-only blueberry jam	125 mL

Put 8 oz. (80 mL) of blueberries in a food processor or blender along with the cornstarch and jam. Process until the mixture is liquid and well blended. Pour into a small saucepan. Cook over low heat, stirring constantly until thickened and bright. Remove from the heat. Add the reserved blueberries. Stir. Serve warm or cold. Keeps well in the refrigerator.

Yield: 1½ C (375 mL) **Exchange:** ½ fruit
Each T (15 mL) contains:
Calories: 56 Fiber: 0.2 g
Sodium: trace Cholesterol: 4 mg

Strawberry Topping

Serve this over frozen yogurt, angel food cake, sponge cake, crêpes, or even cream puffs!

2 (16 oz.)pkgs	frozen, sliced strawberries, no sugar added, thawed	2 (465 mL) pkgs
5 t	cornstarch	50 mL
½ C	fruit-only strawberry jam	125 mL

Drain one of the packages of frozen strawberries. Set aside. Put the other package, cornstarch, and jam in a blender or food processor. Process until liquid is well blended. Pour into a small saucepan. Cook over heat, stirring constantly, until thickened and bright. Remove from heat. Add drained strawberries. Stir. Serve warm or cold. Keeps well in the refrigerator.

Yield: 4 C (64 T)   **Exchange:** free
1 T (15 mL) contains:
Calories: 24   Fiber: trace
Sodium: trace   Cholesterol: 0.5 mg

Cherry Topping

This can top Icy Grapes or any dessert that needs some extra pizzazz.

1 (14.5oz) can	pitted cherries (packed in water only)	1 (415 mL) can
2 T	cornstarch	60 mL
1 T	cherry-flavored brandy (optional)	15 mL
1 t	aspartame	5 mL
a few drops	red food coloring (optional)	a few drops

Drain water off cherries and put ¼ C liquid in a saucepan with cornstarch. Add brandy. Stir over medium heat for a few minutes, stirring with a wire whisk, until it boils and becomes thickened. Remove from heat; add cherries, aspartame and red food coloring, if desired.

Yield: 6 servings   **Exchange:** ½ fruit
Each serving contains:
Calories: 39   Fiber: 0
Sodium: trace   Cholesterol: 0

Crunchy Topping for Iced Desserts

Yes, it is unusual to top desserts with chickpeas. But they're good, and they're rich in fiber!

1 (15 oz) can	chickpeas	1 (425 g) can
6 pkts	concentrated acesulfame-K	6 pkts
4 t	cinnamon	20 mL
1 t	vanilla extract	5 mL
½ t	nutmeg	2 mL
2 T	measures-like-sugar aspartame	30 mL

Drain the liquid from a can of chickpeas and pour the chickpeas into a saucepan. Cover with water and add acesulfame-K, cinnamon, and vanilla extract. Cook over medium heat for half an hour. Let cool. Drain off the cooking liquid. Place the chickpeas in a single layer on a large flat pan or cookie sheet with a rim, a pan that has been coated with non-stick cooking spray. Bake in a preheated 375°F (190°C) oven for an hour. Then combine the nutmeg and aspartame in a paper bag. Put the chickpeas into the bag and shake to coat them. Store in an airtight container in the refrigerator for serving over iced desserts.

Yield: 2 C (500 mL) or 8 servings   **Exchange:** free
2 T (30 mL) contain:
Calories: 21.75   Fiber: trace
Sodium: 54 mg   Cholesterol: 0

Maple Walnut Topping

This is wonderful over frozen desserts. Be careful to note what form of sweetener is in various syrups.

1 C	pancake syrup with no sugar added	250 mL
1 t	butter-flavored extract	5 mL
½ t	concentrated aspartame	2 mL
⅓ C	walnuts, chopped	90 mL

Combine all the ingredients in a small bowl and whisk together. To serve hot, heat, but only briefly (for a few seconds) in a microwave oven.

Yield: 21 servings per 1⅓ C (340 mL) **Exchange:** free
1 serving contains:
Calories: 18   Fiber: 1 g
Sodium: 20 mg   Cholesterol: 0

Nonfat Whipped Topping

Make this just before serving. Karin likes to chill it during dinnertime.

⅓ C	nonfat milk	90 mL
⅓ C	instant dry milk solids	90 mL
2 t	fructose	10 mL
½–1 t	vanilla	2–5 mL

Put a bowl with nonfat milk in the freezer until ice crystals begin to form, about 15–20 minutes. Chill the beaters. With an electric mixer at high speed, beat the nonfat dry milk solids into the nonfat milk for 2 minutes, until soft peaks form. Add the fructose and vanilla extract and beat about 2 additional minutes. Use within 20 minutes to avoid the cream separating.

Yield: 24 servings   **Exchange:** free
1 T (15 mL) contains:
Calories: 8   Fiber: 0
Sodium: 10 mg   Cholesterol: trace

Bittersweet Sauce

This is fabulous drizzled over cream puffs or an angel food cake or any time you want a not-too-sweet chocolaty sauce.

3 T	unsweetened cocoa powder	45 mL
1 T	flour	15 mL
1½ C	nonfat milk	375 mL
2 T	margarine or butter (optional)	30 mL
3 pkts	concentrated acesulfame-K	3 pkts
1 t	vanilla extract	5 mL

Combine the cocoa and flour in the top of a double boiler. Add the milk slowly, stirring until the mixture is free of lumps. Cook over boiling water, stirring until the mixture is thick and smooth. Remove from the heat and stir in the margarine or butter. Let cool for 15 minutes. Add the acesulfame-K and vanilla extract. Stir. Serve.

Yield: 24 servings   **Exchange:** free
1 T (15 mL) contains:
Calories: 8   Fiber: trace
Sodium: 12 mg   Cholesterol: trace

Chocolate Sauce

Very good over any dessert.

2 T	unsweetened cocoa powder	30 mL
2 T	cornstarch	30 mL
pinch	salt (optional)	pinch
¾ C	water	190 mL
1 oz.	nonfat cream cheese	30 g
2 t	vanilla extract	10 mL
2 t	concentrated aspartame	10 mL

Combine the first three ingredients in a saucepan. Add the water and cream cheese. Use a wire whisk to stir, and cook until thickened. Turn off the heat. Add the vanilla extract and aspartame. Stir well to combine.

Yield: 1 C (250 mL)   **Exchange:** free
1 T (15 mL) contains:
Calories: 7   Fiber: 0
Sodium: 13 mg   Cholesterol: trace

Rum Sauce

This adds a rich taste to plain puddings, plain frozen desserts, or over plain cake.

1 C	nonfat frozen yogurt, no sugar added	250 mL
1 t	rum extract	5 mL

Allow the yogurt to defrost. Whisk in the rum extract until it's well blended and smooth. Store in the refrigerator.

Yield: 1 C (250 mL)   **Exchange:** free
1 T (15 mL) contains:
Calories: 10   Fiber: 0
Sodium: 9 mg   Cholesterol: 0

Exchange Lists for Meal Planning

Exchange lists are foods listed together because they are alike. Each serving of a food has about the same amount of carbohydrate, protein, fat, and calories as the other foods on that list. That is why any food on a list can be "exchanged" or traded for any other food on the same list. For example, you can trade the slice of bread you might eat for breakfast for one-half cup of cooked cereal. Each of these foods equals one starch choice.

Exchange Lists
Foods are listed with their serving sizes, which are usually measured after cooking. When you begin, you should measure the size of each serving. This may help you learn to "eyeball" correct serving sizes.

The following chart shows the amount of nutrients in one serving from each list.

Groups/Lists	Carbohydrate (grams)	Protein (grams)	Fat (grams)	Calories
Carbohydrate Group				
Starch	15	3	1 or less	80
Fruit	15	—	—	60
Milk				
Skim	12	8	0-3	90
Low-fat	12	8	5	120
Whole	12	8	8	150
Other carbohydrates	15	varies	varies	varies
Vegetables	5	2	—	25
Meat and Meat Substitute Group				
Very lean	—	7	0-1	35
Lean	—	7	3	55
Medium-fat	—	7	5	75
High-fat	—	7	8	100
Fat Group	—	—	5	45

The exchange lists provide you with a lot of food choices (foods from the basic food groups, foods with added sugars, free foods, combination foods, and fast foods). This gives you variety in your meals. Several foods, such as dried beans and peas, bacon, and peanut butter, are on two lists. This gives you flexibility in putting your meals together. Whenever you choose new foods or vary your meal plan, monitor your blood glucose to see how these different foods affect your blood glucose level.

Most foods in the Carbohydrate group have about the same amount of carbohydrate per serving. You can exchange starch, fruit, or milk choices in your meal plan. Vegetables are in this group but contain only about 5 grams of carbohydrate.

Starch List

Cereals, grains, pasta, breads, crackers, snacks, starchy vegetables, and cooked dried beans, peas, and lentils are starches. In general, one starch is:
- ½ cup of cereal, grain, pasta, or starchy vegetable,
- 1 ounce of a bread product, such as 1 slice of bread,
- ¾ to 1 ounce of most snack foods. (Some snack foods may also have added fat.)

Nutrition Tips
1. Most starch choices are good sources of B vitamins.
2. Foods made from whole grains are good sources of fiber.
3. Dried beans and peas are a good source of protein and fiber.

Selection Tips
1. Choose starches made with little fat as often as you can.
2. Starchy vegetables prepared with fat count as one starch and one fat.
3. Bagels or muffins can be 2, 3, or 4 ounces in size, and can, therefore, count as 2, 3, or 4 starch choices. Check the size you eat.
4. Dried beans, peas, and lentils are also found on the Meat and Meat Substitutes list.
5. Most of the serving sizes are measured after cooking.
6. Always check the Nutrition Facts on the food label.

One starch exchange equals 15 grams carbohydrate, 3 grams protein, 0–1 grams fat, and 80 calories.

Bread

Bagel	½ (1 oz)
Bread, reduced calorie	2 slices (1½ oz)
Bread, white, whole wheat, pumpernickel, rye	1 slice (1 oz)
Bread sticks, crisp, 4 in. long x ½ in	2 (⅔ oz)
English muffin	½
Hot dog or hamburger bun	½ (1 oz)
Pita, 6 in. across	½
Roll, plain, small	1 (1 oz)
Raisin bread, unfrosted	1 slice (1 oz)
Tortilla, corn, 6 in. across	1
Tortilla, flour, 7–8 in. across	1
Waffle, 4 ½ in. square, reduced-fat	1

Cereals and Grains

Bran cereals	½ cup
Bulgur	½ cup
Cereals	½ cup
Cereals, unsweetened, ready-to-eat	¾ cup
Cornmeal (dry)	3 Tbsp
Couscous	⅓ cup
Flour (dry)	3 Tbsp
Granola, low-fat	¼ cup
Grape-Nuts	¼ cup
Grits	½ cup
Kasha	½ cup
Millet	¼ cup
Muesli	¼ cup
Oats	½ cup
Pasta	½ cup
Puffed cereal	1½ cups
Rice milk	½ cup
Rice, white or brown	⅓ cup
Shredded Wheat	½ cup
Sugar-frosted cereal	½ cup
Wheat germ	3 Tbsp

Starchy Vegetables

Baked beans	⅓ cup
Corn	½ cup
Corn on cob, medium	1 (5 oz)
Mixed vegetables with corn, peas, or pasta	1 cup

Peas, green	½ cup	Lima beans	⅔ cup
Plantain	½ cup	Lentils	½ cup
Potato, baked or boiled	1 small (3 oz)	Miso 🔺	3 Tbsp
Potato, mashed	½ cup		

Squash, winter (acorn, butternut)	1 cup
Yam, sweet potato, plain	½ cup

Starchy Foods Prepared with Fat
(*Count as 1 starch exchange, plus 1 fat exchange.*)

Crackers and Snacks

Animal crackers	8	Biscuit, 2½ in. across	1
Graham crackers, 2½ in. square	3	Chow mein noodles	½ cup
Matzoh	¾ oz	Corn bread, 2 in. cube	1 (2 oz)
Melba toast	4 slices	Crackers, round butter type	6
Oyster crackers	24	Croutons	1 cup
Popcorn (popped, no fat added		French-fried potatoes	16–25 (3 oz)
or low-fat microwave)	3 cups	Granola	¼ cup
Pretzels	¾ oz	Muffin, small	1 (1½ oz)
Rice cakes, 4 in. across	2	Pancake, 4 in. across	2
Saltine-type crackers	6	Popcorn, microwave	3 cups
Snack chips, fat-free		Sandwich crackers,	
(tortilla, potato)	15–20 (¾ oz)	cheese or peanut butter filling	3
Whole-wheat crackers,		Stuffing, bread (prepared)	⅓ cup
no fat added	2–5 (¾ oz)	Taco shell, 6 in. across	2
		Waffle, 4½ in. square	1

Dried Beans, Peas, and Lentils
(*Count as 1 starch exchange, plus 1 very lean meat exchange.*)

Whole-wheat crackers,
fat added	4–6 (1 oz)

Beans and peas (garbanzo, pinto,
kidney, white, split, black-eyed)	½ cup

🔺 = 400 mg or more of sodium per serving.

Some food you buy uncooked will weigh less after you cook it. Starches often swell in cooking, so a small amount of uncooked starch will become a much larger amount of cooked food. The following table shows some of the changes.

Food (Starch Group)	Uncooked	Cooked
Oatmeal	3 Tbsp	½ cup
Cream of Wheat	2 Tbsp	½ cup
Grits	3 Tbsp	½ cup
Rice	2 Tbsp	⅓ cup
Spaghetti	¼ cup	½ cup
Noodles	⅓ cup	½ cup
Macaroni	¼ cup	½ cup
Dried beans	¼ cup	½ cup
Dried peas	¼ cup	½ cup
Lentils	3 Tbsp	½ cup

Fruit List

Fresh, frozen, canned, and dried fruits and fruit juices are on this list. In general, one fruit exchange is:
• 1 small to medium fresh fruit,
• ½ cup of canned or fresh fruit or fruit juice,
• ¼ cup of dried fruit.

Nutrition Tips
1. Fresh, frozen, and dried fruits have about 2 grams of fiber per choice. Fruit juices contain very little fiber.
2. Citrus fruits, berries, and melons are good sources of vitamin C.

Selection Tips
1. Count ½ cup cranberries or rhubarb sweetened with sugar substitutes as free foods.
2. Read the Nutrition Facts on the food label. If one serving has more than 15 grams of carbohydrate, you will need to adjust the size of the serving you eat or drink.
3. Portion sizes for canned fruits are for the fruit and a small amount of juice.
4. Whole fruit is more filling than fruit juice and may be a better choice.
5. Food labels for fruits may contain the words "no sugar added" or "unsweetened." This means that no sucrose (table sugar) has been added.
6. Generally, fruit canned in extra light syrup has the same amount of carbohydrate per serving as the "no sugar added" or the juice pack. All canned fruits on the fruit list are based on one of these three types of pack.

One fruit exchange equals 15 grams carbohydrate and 60 calories. The weight includes skin, core, seeds, and rind.

Fruit		
Apple, unpeeled, small	1 (4 oz)	Grapefruit sections, canned ¾ cup
Applesauce, unsweetened	½ cup	Grapes, small 17 (3 oz)
Apples, dried	4 rings	Honeydew melon 1 slice (10 oz)
Apricots, fresh	4 whole (5½ oz)	or 1 cup cubes
Apricots, dried	8 halves	Kiwi 1 (3½ oz)
Apricots, canned	½ cup	Mandarin oranges, canned ¾ cup
Banana, small	1 (4 oz)	Mango, small ½ fruit (5½ oz) or ½ cup
Blackberries	¾ cup	Nectarine, small 1 (5 oz)
Blueberries	¾ cup	Orange, small 1 (6½ oz)
Cantaloupe, small	⅓ melon (11 oz)	Papaya ½ fruit (8 oz) or 1 cup cubes
	or 1 cup cubes	Peach, medium, fresh 1 (6 oz)
Cherries, sweet, fresh	12 (3 oz)	Peaches, canned ½ cup
Cherries, sweet, canned	½ cup	Pear, large, fresh ½ (4 oz)
Dates	3	Pears, canned ½ cup
Figs, fresh	1½ large or 2 medium (3 ½ oz)	Pineapple, fresh ¾ cup
Figs, dried	1½	Pineapple, canned ½ cup
Fruit cocktail	½ cup	Plums, canned ½ cup
Grapefruit, large	½ (11 oz)	Plums, small 2 (5 oz)
		Prunes, dried 3

Raisins	2 Tbsp	Cranberry juice cocktail	⅓ cup
Raspberries	1 cup	Cranberry juice cocktail,	
Strawberries	1¼ cup whole berries	reduced-calorie	1 cup
Tangerines, small	2 (8 oz)	Fruit juice blends, 100% juice	⅓ cup
Watermelon	1 slice (13½ oz)	Grape juice	⅓ cup
	or 1¼ cup cubes	Grapefruit juice	½ cup
		Orange juice	½ cup
Fruit Juice		Pineapple juice	½ cup
Apple juice/cider	½ cup	Prune juice	⅓ cup

Milk List

Different types of milk and milk products are on this list. Cheeses are on the Meat list and cream and other dairy fats are on the Fat list. Based on the amount of fat they contain, milks are divided into skim/very low-fat milk, low-fat milk, and whole milk. One choice of these includes:

	Carbohydrate (grams)	Protein (grams)	Fat (grams)	Calories
Skim/very low-fat	12	8	0–3	90
Low-fat	12	8	5	120
Whole	12	8	8	150

Nutrition Tips

1. Milk and yogurt are good sources of calcium and protein. Check the food label.
2. The higher the fat content of milk and yogurt, the greater the amount of saturated fat and cholesterol. Choose lower-fat varieties.
3. For those who are lactose intolerant, look for lactose-reduced or lactose-free varieties of milk.

Selection Tips

1. One cup equals 8 fluid ounces or ½ pint.
2. Nondairy creamers are on the Free Foods list.
3. Look for rice milk on the Starch list.

One milk exchange equals 12 grams carbohydrate and 8 grams protein.

Skim and Very Low-Fat Milk
(0–3 grams fat per serving)

Skim milk	1 cup
½% milk	1 cup
1% milk	1 cup
Nonfat or low-fat buttermilk	1 cup
Evaporated skim milk	½ cup
Nonfat dry milk	⅓ cup dry
Plain nonfat yogurt	¾ cup
Nonfat or low-fat fruit-flavored yogurt sweetened with aspartame or with a nonnutritive sweetener	1 cup

Low-Fat Milk *(5 grams fat per serving)*

2% milk	1 cup
Plain low-fat yogurt	¾ cup
Sweet acidophilus milk	1 cup

Whole Milk *(8 grams fat per serving)*

Whole milk	1 cup
Evaporated whole milk	½ cup
Goat's milk	1 cup
Kefir	1 cup

Meat and Meat Substitutes List

Meat and meat substitutes that contain both protein and fat are on this list. In general, one meat exchange is:
• 1 oz meat, fish, poultry, or cheese,
• ½ cup dried beans.
Based on the amount of fat they contain, meats are divided into very lean, lean, medium-fat, and high-fat lists. This is done so you can see which ones contain the least amount of fat. One ounce (one exchange) of each of these includes:

	Carbohydrate (grams)	Protein (grams)	Fat (grams)	Calories
Very lean	0	7	0–1	35
Lean	0	7	3	55
Medium-fat	0	7	5	75
High-fat	0	7	8	100

Nutrition Tips

1. Choose very lean and lean meat choices whenever possible. Items from the high-fat group are high in saturated fat, cholesterol, and calories and can raise blood cholesterol levels.
2. Meats do not have any fiber.
3. Dried beans, peas, and lentils are good sources of fiber.
4. Some processed meats, seafood, and soy products may contain carbohydrate when consumed in large amounts. Check the Nutrition Facts on the label to see if the amount is close to 15 grams. If so, count it as a carbohydrate choice as well as a meat choice.

Selection Tips

1. Weigh meat after cooking and removing bones and fat. Four ounces of raw meat is equal to 3 ounces of cooked meat. Some examples of meat portions are:
   • 1 ounce cheese = 1 meat choice and is about the size of a l-inch cube
   • 2 ounces meat = 2 meat choices, such as 1 small chicken leg or thigh, ½ cup cottage cheese or tuna
   • 3 ounces meat = 3 meat choices and is about the size of a deck of cards, such as 1 medium pork chop, 1 small hamburger, ½ a whole chicken breast, 1 unbreaded fish fillet
2. Limit your choices from the high-fat group to three times per week or less.
3. Most grocery stores stock Select and Choice grades of meat. Select grades of meat are the leanest meats. Choice grades contain a moderate amount of fat, and Prime cuts of meat have the highest amount of fat. Restaurants usually serve Prime cuts of meat.
4. "Hamburger" may contain added seasoning and fat, but ground beef does not.
5. Read labels to find products that are low in fat and cholesterol (5 grams or less of fat per serving).
6. Dried beans, peas, and lentils are also found on the Starch list.
7. Peanut butter, in smaller amounts, is also found on the Fats list.
8. Bacon, in smaller amounts, is also found on the Fats list.

Meal Planning Tips
1. Bake, roast, broil, grill, poach, steam, or boil these foods rather than frying.
2. Place meat on a rack so the fat will drain off during cooking.
3. Use a nonstick spray and a nonstick pan to brown or fry foods.
4. Trim off visible fat before or after cooking.
5. If you add flour, bread crumbs, coating mixes, fat, or marinades when cooking, ask your dietitian how to count it in your meal plan.

Lean Meat and Substitutes List

One exchange equals 0 grams carbohydrate,
7 grams protein, 3 grams fat, and 55 calories.

One lean meat exchange is equal to any one of the following items.

Beef: USDA Select or Choice grades of lean beef trimmed of fat, such as round, sirloin, and flank steak; tenderloin; roast (rib, chuck, rump); steak (T-bone, porterhouse, cubed); ground round — 1 oz

Pork: Lean pork, such as fresh ham; canned, cured, or boiled ham; Canadian bacon; ◣ tenderloin, center loin chop — 1 oz

Lamb: Roast, chop, leg — 1 oz

Veal: Lean chop, roast — 1 oz

Poultry: Chicken, turkey (dark meat, no skin), chicken white meat (with skin), domestic duck or goose (well-drained of fat, no skin) — 1 oz

Fish:
Herring (uncreamed or smoked) — 1 oz
Oysters — 6 medium

Salmon (fresh or canned), catfish — 1 oz
Sardines (canned) — 2 medium
Tuna (canned in oil, drained) — 1 oz

Game: Goose (no skin), rabbit — 1 oz

Cheese:
4.5%-fat cottage cheese — ¼ cup
Grated Parmesan — 2 Tbsp
Cheeses with 3 grams or less fat per ounce — 1 oz

Other:
Hot dogs with 3 grams or less fat per ounce ◣ — 1½ oz
Processed sandwich meat with 3 grams or less fat per ounce, such as turkey pastrami or kielbasa — 1 oz
Liver, heart (high in cholesterol) — 1 oz

◣ = 400 mg or more of sodium per exchange.

Fat List

Fats are divided into three groups, based on the main type of fat they contain: monounsaturated, polyunsaturated, and saturated. Small amounts of monounsaturated and polyunsaturated fats in the foods we eat are linked with good health benefits. Saturated fats are linked with heart disease and cancer. In general, one fat exchange is:
• 1 teaspoon of regular margarine or vegetable oil,
• 1 tablespoon of regular salad dressings.

Nutrition Tips
1. All fats are high in calories. Limit serving sizes for good nutrition and health.
2. Nuts and seeds contain small amounts of fiber, protein, and magnesium.
3. If blood pressure is a concern, choose fats in the unsalted form to help lower sodium intake, such as unsalted peanuts.

Selection Tips

1. Check the Nutrition Facts on food labels for serving sizes. One fat exchange is based on a serving size containing 5 grams of fat.
2. When selecting regular margarine, choose those with liquid vegetable oil as the first ingredient. Soft margarines are not as saturated as stick margarines. Soft margarines are healthier choices. Avoid those listing hydrogenated or partially hydrogenated fat as the first ingredient.
3. When selecting low-fat margarines, look for liquid vegetable oil as the second ingredient. Water is usually the first ingredient.
4. When used in smaller amounts, bacon and peanut butter are counted as fat choices. When used in larger amounts, they are counted as high-fat meat choices.
5. Fat-free salad dressings are on the Free Foods list.
6. See the Free Foods list for nondairy coffee creamers, whipped topping, and fat-free products, such as margarines, salad dressings, mayonnaise, sour cream, cream cheese, and nonstick cooking spray.

Monounsaturated Fats List

One fat exchange equals 5 grams fat and 45 calories.

Avocado, medium	⅛ (1 oz)
Oil (canola, olive, peanut)	1 tsp
Olives: ripe (black)	8 large
green, stuffed ◣	10 large
Nuts	
almonds, cashews	6 nuts
mixed (50% peanuts)	6 nuts
peanuts	10 nuts
pecans	4 halves
Peanut butter, smooth or crunchy	2 tsp
Sesame seeds	1 Tbsp
Tahini paste	2 tsp

Polyunsaturated Fats List

One fat exchange equals 5 grams fat and 45 calories.

Margarine: stick, tub, or squeeze	1 tsp
lower-fat	
(30% to 50% vegetable oil)	1 Tbsp
Mayonnaise: regular	1 tsp
reduced-fat	1 Tbsp
Nuts, walnuts, English	4 halves
Oil (corn, safflower, soybean)	1 tsp
Salad dressing: regular ◣	1 Tbsp
reduced-fat	2 Tbsp
Miracle Whip Salad Dressing®: regular	2 tsp
reduced-fat	1 Tbsp

Seeds: pumpkin, sunflower	1 Tbsp

Saturated Fats List*

One fat exchange equals 5 grams of fat and 45 calories.

Bacon, cooked	1 slice (20 slices/lb)
Bacon, grease	1 tsp
Butter: stick	1 tsp
whipped	2 tsp
reduced-fat	1 Tbsp
Chitterlings, boiled	2 Tbsp (½ oz)
Coconut, sweetened, shredded	2 Tbsp
Cream, half and half	2 Tbsp
Cream cheese: regular	1 Tbsp (½ oz)
reduced-fat	2 Tbsp (1 oz)
Fatback or salt pork, *see below*	
Shortening or lard	1 tsp
Sour cream: regular	2 Tbsp
reduced-fat	3 Tbsp

◣ = 400 mg or more sodium per exchange.

Use a piece 1 in. x 1 in. x ¼ in. if you plan to eat the fatback cooked with vegetables. Use a piece 2 in. x 1 in. x ½ in. when eating only the vegetables with the fatback removed.

*Saturated fats can raise blood cholesterol levels.

Free Foods List

A free food is any food or drink that contains less than 20 calories or less than 5 grams of carbohydrate per serving. Foods with a serving size listed should be limited to three servings per day. Be sure to spread them out throughout the day. If you eat all three servings at one time, it could affect your blood glucose level. Foods listed without a serving size can be eaten as often as you like.

Fat-Free or Reduced-Fat Foods

Cream cheese, fat-free	1 Tbsp
Creamers, nondairy, liquid	1 Tbsp.
Creamers, nondairy, powder	2 tsp
Mayonnaise, fat-free	1 Tbsp
Mayonnaise, reduced-fat	1 tsp
Margarine, fat-free	4 Tbsp
Margarine, reduced-fat	1 tsp
Miracle Whip®, nonfat	1 Tbsp
Miracle Whip®, reduced-fat	1 tsp
Nonstick cooking spray	
Salad dressing, fat-free	1 Tbsp
Salad dressing, fat-free, Italian	2 Tbsp
Salsa	¼ cup
Sour cream, fat-free, reduced-fat	1 Tbsp.
Whipped topping, regular or light	2 Tbsp

Sugar-Free or Low-Sugar Foods

Candy, hard, sugar-free	1 candy
Gelatin dessert, sugar-free	
Gelatin, unflavored	
Gum, sugar-free	
Jam or jelly, low-sugar or light	2 tsp
Sugar substitutes	
Syrup, sugar-free	2 Tbsp

Sugar substitutes, alternatives, or replacements that are approved by the Food and Drug Administration (FDA) are safe to use. Common brand names include:

- Equal® (aspartame)
- Sprinkle Sweet® (saccharin)
- Sweet One® (acesulfame K)
- Sweet-10® (saccharin)
- Sugar Twin® (saccharin)
- Sweet'n Low® (saccharin)

Drinks

Bouillon, broth, consommé ◣	
Bouillon or broth, low-sodium	
Carbonated or mineral water	
Cocoa powder, unsweetened	1 Tbsp
Coffee	
Club soda	
Diet soft drinks, sugar-free	
Drink mixes, sugar-free	
Tea	
Tonic water, sugar-free	

Condiments

Catsup	1 Tbsp
Horseradish	
Lemon juice	
Lime juice	
Mustard	
Pickles, dill ◣	1½ large
Soy sauce, regular or light ◣	
Taco sauce	1 Tbsp
Vinegar	

Seasonings

Be careful with seasonings that contain sodium or are salts, such as garlic or celery salt, and lemon pepper.

Flavoring extracts
Garlic
Herbs, fresh or dried
Pimento
Spices
Tabasco® or hot pepper sauce
Wine, used in cooking
Worcestershire sauce

◣ = 400 mg or more of sodium per choice.

INDEX